Other books by Marc Bloom

Cross Country Running

The Marathon

Olympic Gold

The Runner's Bible

Know Your Game (series)

The Miler

Run with the Champions

God on the Starting Line

Young Runners

The Complete Guide to Healthy Running for Kids from 5 to 18

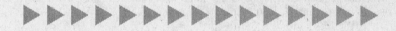

Marc Bloom

A Fireside Book
Published by Simon & Schuster
New York   London   Toronto   Sydney

For Jordana and Max,
future runners

Fireside
A Division of Simon & Schuster, Inc.
1230 Avenue of the Americas
New York, NY 10020

Copyright © 2009 by Marc Bloom

First Fireside trade paperback edition March 2009

FIRESIDE and colophon are registered trademarks of Simon & Schuster, Inc.

For information about special discounts for bulk purchases, please contact Simon & Schuster Special Sales at 1-800-456-6798 or business@simonandschuster.com.

Designed by Carla Jayne Little

Manufactured in the United States of America

10   9   8   7   6   5   4   3   2   1

Library of Congress Cataloging-in-Publication Data

Bloom, Marc.
   Young runners : the complete guide to healthy running for kids from 5 to 18 / Marc Bloom.
      p.   cm.
   "A Fireside Book."
      1. Running—Juvenile literature.   2. Physical fitness—Juvenile literature.   3. Exercise—Juvenile literature.   I. Title.
   GV1061.B57   2009
   613.7'172083—dc22   2008054834

ISBN-13: 978-1-4165-7299-2
ISBN-10   1-4165-7299-6

Contents

Preface

Young Runners: The Rules

When I'm running it's like an obstacle and I just want to break the wall down and push so hard so I can get to the next level and I'm even better and have more challenges.

—SASHA ESTRELLA-JONES, SEVENTH-GRADE RUNNER
AT A BROOKLYN, NEW YORK, MIDDLE SCHOOL

1. All children and teenagers can learn to love running.
2. Running is easy when approached with patience and common sense.
3. Running progress should be gradual over time.
4. Running is done mainly for fun, learning, and good health.
5. Running should not dominate a child's life.
6. Running enjoyment is enhanced with friends and school-mates.
7. Parents who run are the best role models for their children.
8. Children's growth and development must be taken into account.
9. Children approach running differently than adults.
10. Competition should not put undue pressure on running children.

Introduction

The Kids' Running Revolution

I challenge my students. They have to run 3 miles a day even if they're on vacation in Puerto Rico.

—STEVE SLOAN, MIGHTY MILERS COACH AT AN
EAST HARLEM ELEMENTARY SCHOOL, NEW YORK CITY

On a school night in the winter of 1982, I collected my 9-year-old daughter, Allison, and trekked into Manhattan so she could do a speed workout on an indoor track overhanging a gymnasium at Columbia University. Allison was a third grader at the time, had been running on and off for years, and trying to make the finals of the Colgate Women's Games track program in the youngest age group, first through third grade. Her event was the 800 meters and she had the semifinal round coming up. A good race could vault her into the Madison Square Garden final.

We were then living on Staten Island, and I could not locate a nearby indoor track on this particular night—a night I'd assigned for speed. Many desperate phone calls yielded Columbia as the only game in town.

That evening, the university track was filled with adult joggers who marveled at the little girl zipping past them, lap after lap. With stopwatch in hand, I called out times, trying to motivate Allison to perform like a professional. I felt this dedication would firm up her commitment to become a runner and set her on a path of hard work and good values, encourage self-confidence, dispel gender stereotypes and—who knew?—maybe one day land her on the United States Olympic team. I considered Colgate a springboard. We got home around midnight.

Allison ran well in the semis and made the 800 finals, and our whole family turned out for the big day. The 225 finalists were hailed by celebrities including Lena Horne and Willie Mays. The Garden rocked. And in a quiet corner outside the track arena, I prepped Allison with complex strategies on running the tight track against the five other third graders. She looked at me blankly, thinking, I'm sure, *What is Daddy doing to me?*

On my office wall above the computer, I have a photograph of the six girls lined up on the starting line with the gun about to sound. I look at the photo now. Five of the girls appear relaxed, with arms down, hands loose, neutral posture, and mildly focused expressions. Guess which girl looks tense, with hunched shoulders, fists clenched, and a fearful countenance. Allison placed fifth.

THE PURE FUN OF RUNNING

As I came to my senses and let go of the child star mind-set, Allison went on to play soccer, run high school cross-country, and, at 24, complete the New York City Marathon. She and I can laugh about it now, but I was clearly the type of overzealous, foolhardy track parent that irks me today. Before Allison's races that winter, she would say to me at bedtime, "Dad, I'm nervous. What if I don't run a better time?" Even though I was able to catch myself and let Allison choose her own path as a teenager, I cringe when I think of that period now.

I hope *Young Runners* will help readers emphasize the pure fun of running while letting children progress at their own rate, make their own choices, and take competition as a healthy challenge, not a stepping-stone to stardom. We all want the best for our children, but in a distorted educational landscape that stresses test taking above all else, with the plum of marquee college acceptance, it's all too common for parents to consider running one more subject to master, one more opportunity to outdo others, one more vehicle to enhance a child's and family's stature.

In his research on young athletes, Michigan State sports psychologist Daniel Gould, Ph.D., has seen how closely today's parents seem linked to their children's every hit and miss. "Some parents manifest their own childhood athletic dreams through their child," says Gould, "whereas others might be indirectly reinforcing their worth as a parent through their child's success, as in 'My daughter runs a good time and everyone recognizes her and tells me what a good job I am doing as a parent.'"

It's easy to be seduced by such notions, but by the time our younger daughter, Jamie, started out in sports, I knew enough to stay out of the way, more or less. I was finally and permanently put in my place when it was Jamie's turn to run on the high school team. With her teenage disposition craving acceptance in freshman cross-country, she suffered the ultimate embarrassment when I would show up at meets as the resident expert wearing my red woolen hat—the dorkiest hat in creation. That and my high-cut running shorts. Well, it was all over for me, a track dad put out to pasture.

My early zeal might have been satisfied if only my daughters had had friends to run with as children. I knew that peer support and approval could take them far. But their friends did not run. It was not considered cool. There were no PE teachers organizing running groups or much in the way of kids' programs outside of Colgate, which was highly competitive. When Allison was 5, to enable her to run with other children, we had to take her an hour away to Van Cortlandt Park in the Bronx for a kids' cross-country run. She fell asleep in the stroller wearing her race number and missed the event.

KIDS' RUNNING SWEEPS THE NATION

But we are in a new era now, with children's running sweeping the nation. In response to the alarming statistics on childhood obesity that began to make headlines about a decade ago—one-third of children nationwide are currently obese or overweight— a rallying cry went out and the running community responded. Parents, teachers, coaches, physicians, schools, running clubs, running events, and corporate sponsors have come forth to create nothing less than a kids' running revolution, in which almost every community has some form of meaningful children's running going on. It might be a couple of dozen kids running with a parent leader at a community center or thousands of youngsters turning out for a menu of children's races sponsored by a major marathon. There are more than 100,000 children in the Texas-based Marathon Kids school program and 50,000 in the New York Road Runners Foundation school program.

I estimate that well over 1 million youngsters ages 5 to 12 are engaged in running. And with another 1.1 million teenagers running high school track and cross-country—which show the greatest increases in participation of any sports, according to national statistics—we have a historic movement gathering speed that in time could change the health portrait of the nation. Young runners already appear to be stemming the tide of childhood obesity, according to doctors and researchers I spoke with, but since many of the larger programs are fairly new, it's too soon to tell.

Dr. Jennifer Sluder, a pediatrician at Childrens Hospital Los Angeles who's involved with a number of running programs, says when asked about the impact of running on childhood obesity: "Anecdotally, I know it's making a big difference, but, statistically, you have to do a large study over several years. There are some studies under way at the hospital on obesity and exercise and I think we'll have some concrete evidence soon."

The good news is still not good enough. What about the other children, the sedentary and obese kids who make up the sorry statistics from the federal Centers for Disease Control and Prevention? We have, in effect, two societies of children: healthy, active, running kids who populate fields and parks and tracks working up a sweat, and the unhealthy masses with poor diets and expanding waistlines, many hidden from view as indoor spectators glued to computer and television screens. Unfortunately, the active society also has its extreme wing: parents and coaches who resemble the old me, pushing kids too hard and creating another set of alarming statistics regarding children's injury and burnout rates.

As a journalist writing about youth running for decades, I've seen the best and worst. I've been overcome by tears of joy watching children and teens run, run, run for the sweet satisfactions of reaching a goal, completing an arduous task, helping a team, and sharing in a pure and honest endeavor with friends. I've also been moved to tears of sadness seeing young runners imperiled by the demands of an oppressive coach or parent.

DYNAMIC LEADERS SET THE PACE

I hope this book provides a road map for doing the right thing. In probing for the best ways to engage youngsters in running and nurture their interest for the long term, I considered the children's running landscape as new territory to explore and approached it with a hopeful sense of discovery. I wanted to get close to dynamic people in the field. I went to Springfield, Virginia, to see a Healthy School award winner with a robust running program and to Durham, North Carolina, to see a youth track squad led by a pediatric cardiologist, Dr. Brenda Armstrong, who tests team members for blood pressure and lap times. I ventured into Brooklyn, where I grew up, to watch an intermediate school running club practice at a small concrete park, and to New York's Randall's Island, where I ran in high school, to watch a middle school track meet with private schools' entries among the rich and famous. I took in a wonderful kids' running program in my suburban New Jersey community and, in the most gratifying experience of all, followed a local autistic boy who is thriving in middle school track and cross-country.

In addition, I conducted dozens of interviews with parents, teachers, coaches, school administrators, youth program coordinators, doctors, sports psychologists, sports medicine specialists, and young runners of all ages. I've also known countless people in the field and seen hundreds of youth running events over the years. All this has helped me formulate what I feel are the best methods for getting more kids running and getting them moving in smarter and healthier ways, to enhance the kids' running revolution and make further dents in childhood obesity.

Kids experience the transforming power of running as much as adults do, and in their innocence they can gain even more, if we let them progress at their own pace. "Physical activity like running can improve every aspect of a child's life, from socialization to academic work to disease prevention," says Dr. Bill Roberts, a family practice physician in Minneapolis who is past president of the American College of Sports Medicine and medical director of the Twin Cities Marathon. "Their hearts pump stronger, blood volume goes up, and they maintain lean muscle mass." Fit children can achieve extraordinary levels of heart functioning, according to Dr. Armstrong. From her tests of the runners she coaches, she finds that kids have an ejection fraction—the volume of blood put out by the left ventricle when the heart contracts—close to that of the most highly trained athletes, such as competitive swimmers.

Running children also gain wellness in body, mind, and spirit. Running is holistic, forging better nutrition, relaxation, positive thinking, and seeing the good in yourself and others. Anyone who works with kids will tell you that running empowers youngsters to overcome problems and better understand the world around them. These kids can teach us a thing or two about life, and if you don't believe that, take special note of what some of those in the following chapters have to say.

Running children make for healthier families and a healthier society, and I hope that *Young Runners* offers some ideas on how to raise children to respect their bodies, relate better to others, take responsibility for their actions, and treat people with fairness and decency. Running is a Great Society idea because it not only strengthens the heart but opens the heart. No child left behind? Yes, indeed, when it comes to running.

AT-RISK TEENS GO THE DISTANCE

In the inner cities of California, kids of all stripes are making gains to a remarkable extent in, of all things, marathon running. Now entering its twentieth year, Students Run LA trains middle school and high school youth to run the City of Los Angeles Marathon. Participation has reached over 2,500 with a 95 to 99 percent completion rate, according to one of the program originators, Paul Trapani, whom I spoke with. More than 300 teacher leaders and coaches guide the youngsters from September to the marathon in March. (It was moved to Memorial Day in 2009.) Trapani says that the young marathoners achieve a remarkable 90 percent high school graduation rate (as compared to the 68 percent average for the LA public schools) and that running has had a ripple effect on all aspects of their health and well-being.

Seeing it as a model to help at-risk youth, Philadelphia adopted the LA program as Students Run Philly Style in 2005, targeting neighborhoods with the highest incidence of drug abuse, asthma, and other health issues. That first year, 125 youngsters participated, all new runners, training from March to November for the Philadelphia Marathon and Half-Marathon with the Broad Street 10-Miler in May en route. At a year-end celebration, says program director Heather McDanel, "a 14-year-old girl came onstage and said she used to just watch TV and was shy and the program changed her life." Another student, a 16-year-old boy, participated while undergoing chemotherapy for cancer.

Another winning concept adopted throughout the country is the Texas-based Marathon Kids program, created by Kay Morris in 1995 and now serving more than 100,000 children from kindergarten through fifth grade throughout Texas, with new affiliates in California and Maryland and plans to open in Chicago. It's a run-walk-nutrition program with kids running a quarter mile or half mile to accumulate at least 25 miles in six months; then they run a climactic 1.2 miles en masse to total 26.2 miles—a "marathon." Morris says they target children most in need and that the completion rate is 83 percent. Students keep "fuel logs" of fruits and vegetables consumed and are given 26.2 healthy things to do over the summer.

Children's advocates such as Morris understand that when running programs embrace kids' education as a whole, teach values, and stress lifestyle changes pertaining to nutrition and family, they will be most effective and long-lasting. These program leaders are helping to create better communities.

A similar holistic approach was adopted by the GO! St. Louis Marathon's "Read, Right and Run" program for kindergartners through eighth graders, which has grown from 400 participants in 2001 to 3,000 in 2008, according to director Nancy Lieberman. Older students in middle school do a 5K as their final run. "Read" requires reading twenty-six books. "Right" requires twenty-six good deeds such as tutoring younger children or helping out at Ronald McDonald House. "It's contagious," says Lieberman. On the celebratory race day in April, when the kids line up, "you can't hold them back." The event has added a summer track meet series for kids, will soon train high school students for a half-marathon, and has other events for young children, including a Diaper Dash.

Diaper Dash is practically a circuit. Credit for the original probably goes to the Medtronic Twin Cities Marathon, whose own version has infants crawling in a big circle on the grounds of the Minnesota state capitol. The event, in October, also features a Toddler Trot, among other kids' events, with total participation up to 3,665. "The young kids always want to run more," says Sandy Unger, Medtronic youth program and community outreach manager.

WEB PROGRAMS FUEL INTEREST

The pace of program growth has been accelerated by the Internet. The Web-based Big Sur Marathon Just Run program, begun in the 2004–5 school term, now has about 7,000 children in seventy schools in Monterey County with a Just Run Across the USA component featuring participants in at least fourteen states. Kids log and track mileage, offer running ideas that are posted, and perform good deeds, another concept that is catching on.

Just Run is one of many children's programs nationwide indicating positive health gains in a short time. In 2007, test scores for fifth, seventh, and ninth graders in the five Monterey schools that are part of Just Run showed an increase from 58 percent to 81 percent in the proportion of students passing the Fitnessgram Pacer Test, a measure of aerobic fitness. At the same time, the

eight county schools not in the program saw a drop in those passing from 59 percent to 47 percent, according to Just Run founder
Mike Dove.

And so from the Monterey Peninsula to the Feelin' Good
Mileage Club in Flint, Michigan; from the Fit for Life Challenge
in Richmond, Virginia, to the Fit for Bloomsday program in Spokane, Washington; from the Marine Corps Marathon Healthy
Kids Fun Run in Washington, D.C., to the Smile Mile in Winter
Park, Florida; from the Many Milers Club in Burlington, Vermont, to the Peachtree Junior in Atlanta, Georgia, there are Diaper Dashes, Toddler Trots, Student Sprints, Miles of Smiles,
uphill and downhill races, track and cross-country, road runs and
even marathons propelling kids of all ages, both boys and girls, as
well as those hard-to-motivate teens, to move, move, move, keep
moving, for fun, health, and the greater good.

Seeking to create awareness, provide funding, and give youngsters a running outlet, Nike sponsors a nationwide 5K Run for
Kids program with events in eight cities and over 2,000 young
participants, in addition to several thousand adults. Proceeds
from entry fees are donated to local school physical education
and athletic programs, and according to Nike, over $1 million
has been raised so far. The events offer kids' training runs for
preparation and a one-mile run in addition to the 5K.

The most ambitious undertaking of all is in New York City.
The New York Road Runners, which has led almost every important running movement since the early days of Fred Lebow,
serves more than 50,000 children in the five boroughs and other
cities with several running programs under the auspices of the
New York Road Runners Foundation. With an annual budget of
$5.25 million and a full-time staff of eighteen plus more than
forty part-timers, the foundation has more than 100 elementary
schools in the five boroughs in its Mighty Milers program, another sixty-plus middle schools in its Young Runners program,
and a City Sports for Kids track program.

RUNNING A MILLION MILES IN
NEW YORK AND BEYOND

"Our model is 'train and support,'" says New York Road Runners Foundation executive director Cliff Sperber. The club targets school populations in need, trains site coordinators, gives workout schedules, provides supplies and equipment, offers abundant incentives, has field managers observe team practices, and is allied with key operatives at the city's Board of Education and Department of Health. Their goal is at least a million miles covered in a school term by all participants, including a division in Cape Town, South Africa. Each child has a personalized Web page to keep track of mileage and view the progress of other schools as well. "It's a great tool for goal setting and motivation and for teachers to use in academic integration," says Sperber. "Kids can log in anywhere."

One teacher who can't personally benefit from the Web element but is perhaps the most successful Mighty Miler coach of all is Steve Sloan, 53, of Public School 102 in East Harlem. Sloan is legally blind and has been since birth. His mother died when he was 3, and Sloan grew up in group homes, unable to read at 13. A social worker rescued him, and Sloan hasn't looked back since. A PE teacher for twenty-three years, he has the whole school—345 students, the most in any one program—running four to five times a week on a nearby track. He runs on the track himself every morning before school. On weekends, he runs 3 miles from his Bronx home to a YMCA, where he swims and lifts weights.

Isn't it dangerous for a blind man to run through the Bronx streets unattended?

Sloan's reply: "Well, everything is dangerous for me."

I ask him if there is any way he can keep kids running when they're not in school. He replies that he's working on it. In 2008, Sloan began a pilot program he calls "masters," in which his students were given a summer training schedule to run up to 3 miles a day five to six days a week—on the honor system but with parents signing a daily mileage chart, like a report card. "I challenge my students," Sloan says. "They have to run 3 miles a day, even if they're on vacation in Puerto Rico."

The extent to which children continue running when not supervised, and whether they remain active and sustain a healthy lifestyle in later years, are issues under review as kids' programs mature and lend themselves to follow-up assessments. Marathon Kids and Girls on the Run have studies under way. The preeminent sports scientists Steve Blair and Russ Pate of the University of South Carolina are doing new work in this area. The Twin Cities Marathon is collecting research on the teenagers who have run the event over the years, to see if their injury-free efforts hold up over time.

In the meantime, I'm conducting my own study in my older daughter's backyard. Allison, still running in her mid-30s, is now the mother of our two grandchildren. The older one, 6-year-old Jordana, runs from tree to tree as I coax her to complete the Jordana Loop. Sometimes we do it together. I let her stop and start as she wishes, kick a ball, tumble onto the grass, and chase her little brother. It's hard to say if she will really take an interest in running, but just in case, I've already checked out the high school team.

Marc Bloom
Marlboro, New Jersey
July 2008

1

Running with a Head Start

The single most important health issue for pediatricians in this country today is overweight children.
— ASSERTION BY AN AMERICAN ACADEMY OF PEDIATRICS PHYSICIAN IN 1990

While the kids' running revolution is new, many of its ideas started taking shape two decades ago with the growing evidence of childhood obesity and the increasing number of unhealthy-looking young people in our midst.

For many of us it first came to our notice when we saw overweight kids with their overweight parents walking in the mall. Some of these people were so heavy, indeed obese, that they seemed to totter down the corridors. For me, the most arresting images came at the YMCA where I swim. I would see boys of 8 or 9 coming into the pool with the blubbery midsections associated with middle age. What had happened to the skinny kids whose ribs showed through their skin like an accordion? I wondered how parents could allow their children to become overweight and how we as a society could let that happen. At least these boys were swimming. But whatever number of laps they were doing, it was clearly not enough to overcome the ravages of a high-calorie, high-fat diet. And what about the majority of kids who were not getting any exercise at all?

Even then, this trend was considered a potential health crisis. A 1990 *New York Times Magazine* story, "Today's Kids Turn Off Fitness," by Carin Rubenstein, reported on an analysis of four national studies of 22,000 children by Steven Gortmaker, a professor of sociology at the Harvard University School of Public Health, and Dr. William H. Dietz, a specialist in pediatric nutrition at Tufts University Medical School. Findings showed that between 1963 and 1980, obesity had increased 54 percent in 6-to-11-year-olds and 39 percent in 12-to-17-year-olds. Dietz, currently director of the Centers for Disease Control and Prevention (CDC) Division of Nutrition and Physical Activity, said then that we could expect obese children to become obese adults. The same article quoted Dr. Robert Mendelson, speaking for the American Academy of Pediatrics, as saying, "The single most important health issue for pediatricians in this country today is overweight children." Indeed, out-of-shape, overweight youngsters were starting to show signs of "adult" diseases such as type 2 diabetes, hypertension, and heart disease.

Today, according to the latest CDC surveys, 60 percent of overweight children have at least one risk factor for cardiovascular disease. Indeed, a study presented at the 2008 American Heart Association conference found that the thickness of artery walls of children and teenagers who are obese or have high cholesterol, according to the *New York Times*, resembled the thickness of artery walls of an average 45-year-old.

EARLY YOUTH FITNESS CRUSADE STUNTED

But the origins of childhood obesity go back even further, according to a 1983 *Sports Illustrated* article, whose subtitle asserted, "For most of our citizens, especially young ones, the physical fitness boom is a bust." For adults, as the *Sports Illustrated* story by Jerry Kirshenbaum and Robert Sullivan indicated, a fit lifestyle was adopted mainly by the well-heeled and had not reached the lunch-bucket crowd. For kids, the youth fitness crusade begun in the 1950s by President Dwight Eisenhower—a movement propelled in part by national pride and Cold War assertiveness—had petered out. In 1956, as a result of fitness tests showing American youth lagging far behind kids of other nations, Ike had created the President's Council on Youth Fitness, which in 1963 became the President's Council on Physical Fitness and Sports.

But eventually—as school PE classes began to be cut back, our car-obsessed culture made walking an anachronism, and the Big Mac attack took off—young recruits at the New York City Police Academy were failing fitness requirements, bicycle sales plummeted, tests of schoolchildren showed increasing evidence of heart disease risk factors, and adults claimed to be fit with leisure activities like bowling or softball. Kirshenbaum and Sullivan wrote, "By all accounts, the typical American adult can't climb a flight of stairs without experiencing shortness of breath."

And that was in 1983. Soon after, in *The Runner* magazine, Don Kardong, a 1976 Olympic marathoner and future president of the Road Runners Clubs of America, wrote on how getting more kids running might stem childhood obesity. Kardong's 1986 article, "Why Johnny *Can* Run," offered some optimism. Parents told of their kids' healthful running, like the California mom who said, "My son has picked up sports and fitness by osmosis. I swim, he swims. I run, he runs." Or the upstate New York mom who said of her daughter's running, "She is not only in excellent physical shape but seems happy and confident." Isolated cases, to be sure, but at least it was something.

The California mother was ahead of her time. A decade later, in a study of the effects of overweight parents on their overweight children, Dr. Robert Whitaker, a pediatric obesity expert at Children's Hospital Medical Center in Cincinnati, found that an obese child between ages 6 and 9 had a 37 percent chance of being an obese adult if neither parent was obese, and a 71 percent chance of being an obese adult if at least one parent was fat.

The message was clear. "Be a good role model. Be active. And be active with your children," Janet Fulton, Ph.D., an epidemiologist with the CDC physical activity division, told me in an interview.

In the mid-1980s, Kardong also found the first stirrings of commitment of adult running clubs to develop kids' events. Most noteworthy were the elementary school runs by the Huntsville Track Club in Alabama, which grew to 3,000 participants at the time. And there was Kardong's own hometown event in Spokane, Washington, the Lilac Bloomsday, a 12-kilometer race with a 12-and-under division that by 1986 had grown to 6,000 youngsters as parents and teachers conducted kids' training clinics around town.

Other than the smiles on kids' faces, was there any concrete evidence that these early attempts at running were good for youngsters' health? A 1985 study of Florida fourth, fifth, and sixth graders by Florida State University researchers Bruce W. Tuchman and J. Scott Hinkle was affirmative. After doing three 30-minute runs per week for twelve weeks during school PE classes, a group of 154 boys and girls had less body fat, lower pulse rates, and greater cardiovascular fitness than a group of kids who did their normal PE program of sports and games.

CHILDHOOD OBESITY TRIPLES IN TWENTY YEARS

How did we travel from these small but significant indications of good things to come in the mid-1980s to the most recent findings, released in 2005 and again in 2008, that during this twenty-year-plus period obesity in children ages 2 to 19 had more than tripled to about 17 percent? These figures are based on data from the National Health and Nutrition Examination Surveys with compilations by the CDC. All along, percentages have been highest in the upper age brackets.

The latest figures, from May 2008, showed a cautious sign of hope, as obesity was said to have plateaued. However, a *New York Times* editorial dismissed the leveling off as superficial. Equal percentages of youngsters, while not quite obese, still weighed enough to be considered at risk. That meant that about one out of every three American children, upward of 25 million, were in danger.

"These kids could need coronary bypass in their 20s," said Kelly Brownell, director of the Yale University Center for Eating and Weight Disorders. Indeed, studies have already shown that obesity and elevated cholesterol levels in young people have led to hardening of the coronary arteries as these people get older. And while the latest Surgeon General's report on smoking and health shows that adult smoking has decreased, teenage smoking has increased, especially among girls.

It's no wonder, then, that a 2005 report in the *New England Journal of Medicine* (*NEJM*) said that for the first time the current generation of children in America may live less healthful lives and have shorter life expectancies than their parents. If childhood obesity is left unchecked, said the *New York Times*, this trend could shorten life span by as much as five years. Type 2 diabetes, heart disease, kidney disease, and cancer are likely to strike people at younger and younger ages. According to the authors of the *NEJM* report, obesity is already shortening average life span by a greater rate than accidents, homicides, and suicides combined.

Measures to stop the childhood obesity tide have grown desperate. According to a 2003 *Time* magazine story, at least a dozen hospitals nationwide are performing gastric bypass surgery—"stomach stapling," so that the body can no longer take in normal amounts of food—on kids. One physician estimated that as many as 250,000 U.S. teenagers may be candidates for the operation. Why cut out thousand-calorie McDonald's milk shakes or take a walk in the park when you can take the magic bullet route the way celebrity TV weatherman Al Roker did? Gastric bypass, a procedure costing $25,000 to $40,000 and causing youngsters to miss a month of school, has risks including blood clots, serious infections, and even death. "You're substituting one potentially life-threatening condition for another," Dr. David Ludwig told *Time* magazine's Christine Gorman.

Referring to candy and soda machines in schools, cutbacks in physical education classes, and supersize portions in fast-food restaurants, Gorman concluded, "If you tried to design an environment that would promote obesity in the greatest number of people in the shortest period you could hardly do better than American pop culture in the past 20 years."

Schools have begun to address their unhealthy lunches, on average about 40 percent fat, according to the U.S. Department of Agriculture. Schools prohibiting junk foods in vending machines increased from 8 to 32 percent from 2000 to 2006, according to a 2007 study published in the *Journal of School Health*. Schools offering salads for lunch have increased, while those offering french fries have decreased. But since a child consumes only 20 percent of calories at school, any progress must be weighed against family meals at home and at fast-food restaurants.

CONTINUITY CRITICAL IN HEALTHY CHOICES

The problem of continuity—what a child does *most* of the time even while engaged in healthy activity *some* of the time—is a key factor in the obesity trend. It's why a sound PE program or regular running won't be enough unless a youngster and his family adopt a healthy lifestyle overall. It's why the physician who works with the Durham Striders youth track team in North Carolina insists on good nutrition and other healthy behavior for entire families.

That takes work, and when it comes to health care, our culture relies mainly on drugs. In a development as desperate as gastric bypass, the Food and Drug Administration in 2003 approved for the first time a weight loss drug for overweight children. Called Xenical (also orlistat), it was approved for 12-to-16-year-olds. The drug was said to block the digestion of one-third of the fat a youngster eats. Considering the amount of fat kids take in, it was hard to imagine the effectiveness of the medication, which comes with various side effects.

While this news barely raised an eyebrow at the time, an American Academy of Pediatrics recommendation in July 2008 that more children as young as 8 be given cholesterol-lowering drugs in hopes of preventing adult heart problems caused a furor. For the most part, the AAP was blasted. But, to be fair, the AAP has routinely emphasized better nutritional practices and exercise for children. However, as the *New York Times* noted, doctors and parents were turning increasingly to drug treatment, according to some experts, "because they find lifestyle changes too difficult to implement or enforce."

In another example of meeting kids where they live, as opposed to effecting potentially long-term health changes, there are now "active" video games that have kids gyrating to instructions on the screen. Any movement is better than nothing, and this idea seems like a modern-day Jane Fonda for kids. But will it have legs? A Mayo Clinic study in 2006 found that some of these games resulted in more calories burned than if youngsters walked on a treadmill.

One game, deemed the latest weapon against childhood obesity, is Dance Dance Revolution, in which youngsters dance on a floor mat to music. Originating in Japan, DDR has become part of schools' physical education curriculum in at least ten states, including West Virginia, which sought to have the game in all of its public schools by 2008. *The New York Times* called this a "small craze." Crazes don't last. In 1987, researching a *New York* magazine story on children's exercise classes in the swankier precincts of Manhattan, I witnessed a preteen aerobics class in which kids danced to "The Loco-Motion." It seemed like a movement was starting. Craze was more like it. And tweens are not teens. What's cool at 12 is usually *verboten* at 16.

There's no end to the wrongheadedness in what constitutes healthy activity for kids. Take the recess battle in Connecticut. In 2007, one school principal banned games such as kickball, soccer, and other "body-banging" activities during the students' twenty-two-minute recess, fearing that bodies, and feelings, might get bruised. Children were encouraged to jump rope or use hula hoops. It's not enough that PE is suffering at many schools. But recess? With other schools also behaving badly, a national campaign, Rescuing Recess, an alliance of education and health organizations, started up. Would recess go the way of the one-room schoolhouse?

Connecticut parents had professional expertise on their side. University of Texas education professor Joe Frost, who's researched children's play for thirty years, told the *New York Times* that the watered-down recess was "terrible, ill-advised and damaging" in denying kids the chance to develop social skills and avoid obesity.

"BUBBLE-WRAPPED" YOUNGSTERS MISS FUN

Overprotection, especially of a child's "self-esteem," is an epidemic just like obesity. Together, they can seem like an unstoppable force. But the smart parents of the Connecticut town did get the principal to relent a bit, allowing supervised, modified, nonscoring kickball twice weekly for the older kids. Still outraged, one father summed up the debacle when he complained to the

Times that youngsters should not have to be "bubble-wrapped" before they could have fun.

Well, not in Arkansas, which, oddly enough, seems to be in the forefront of bold stopgap measures. The state has the highest childhood obesity numbers of any state other than Mississippi, and so Arkansas' 1,139 public schools now issue each student a health report card in the form of body mass index, or BMI, a measurement urged for medical use by the American Academy of Pediatrics. Though controversial and easy to pick on for "stigmatizing" kids, the new policy (which also forbids access to vending machines in elementary schools) at least gives parents a needed reality check. Delaware, Pennsylvania, South Carolina, and Tennessee are among other states using BMI report cards.

A number of surveys of parents' own assessments of their children's well-being indicate that moms and dads are clueless. For example, a 2007 University of Michigan survey of 2,000 parents found that over 40 percent of parents were unaware that their kids were obese. "If families had an accurate perception of the issue, we wouldn't need BMI screening," Dr. David Ludwig, the Boston physician, told the *New York Times* in January 2007.

More hope, if you will, has come out of Arkansas. In 2005, Governor Mike Huckabee, the 2008 Republican presidential candidate who runs marathons and has lost over 100 pounds, joined an even more notable Razorback, former president Bill Clinton, a sometime runner who'd had quadruple heart bypass surgery the previous September, to promote an American Heart Association (AHA) program to fight childhood obesity. Under the banner of the Alliance for a Healthier Generation, the AHA and the William J. Clinton Foundation targeted children, especially those 9 to 13, with the goal of stopping the increase in childhood obesity by 2010 and reversing the trend by 2015. The Let's Just Play Go Healthy Challenge and other programs were set up "to empower kids to take charge of their own health."

The American Heart Association has since received a grant of

close to $20 million from the Robert Wood Johnson Foundation
to expand the AHA Healthy Schools programs "in states with the
highest prevalence of obesity." That has been the biggest single
award thus far from the foundation, which announced in April
2007 a $500 million five-year commitment to reverse childhood
obesity in the United States by 2015.

Coincidentally, the 2005 Huckabee-Clinton announcement
was made at a public school in the Washington Heights section
of Manhattan, practically around the corner from perhaps the
nation's greatest single source of active youth: the New Balance
Track and Field Center. During the winter, upward of 100,000
teenagers from New York and beyond use the facility, which
boasts an Olympic-level track, for practice and competition.

If only that same level of energy and commitment could be
applied elsewhere. Mike Huckabee and Bill Clinton may have
lent their star power to reducing childhood obesity, but barely a
word on the subject was heard during the 2008 presidential campaign. If children were in good shape, the health care crisis would
surely be less of a time bomb. Obese and overweight citizens cost
the United States $117 billion a year in medical bills and lost
productivity, leading to 300,000 deaths a year; of that financial
burden, $14 billion is directly related to childhood obesity.

COMPUTERS AND TV STEAL KIDS' TIME

Few experts face the problems more directly than Dr. Robert
Strauss, head of the Robert Wood Johnson School of Medicine
childhood weight control program in New Brunswick, New Jersey. The synergy between the medical school and the Robert
Wood Johnson Foundation has to be advantageous. In a 2000
study in which he and colleagues studied activity in children ages
10 to 16, Strauss found that kids did basically "nothing" for ten
hours a day and were vigorously active (moving faster than 3.5

miles per hour, a fast walk) an average of only twelve minutes a day. Most of kids' time was spent in front of a TV or computer screen, Strauss said.

"Being inside used to be boring," Strauss told *New York Times* science writer Gina Kolata for her front-page story "While Children Grow Fatter, Experts Search for Solutions." "Now it's exciting."

Another study, in 2008, affirmed Strauss' finding of youngsters' sedentary existence as they enter the teen years. Research financed by the National Institutes of Health, which tracked about 1,000 children nationwide, showed a dramatic shift from three hours of movement a day for a child at age 9 to less than one hour a day by 13.

Those of us of a certain age recall the days when much of our youth was spent pleading with Mom to let us stay outside. In my Brooklyn neighborhood, youngsters were creative geniuses at playing sports on tiny plots of concrete. I knew no one who took a bus to school.

Much childhood obesity could be eliminated if only kids walked to school. A mile walk, with youngsters carrying schoolbooks, would take about forty-five minutes round-trip. That's 75 percent of the sixty minutes of daily exercise now recommended by the CDC. Add a little PE and a bike ride on the weekends, and you've got it. But the newer suburbs barely have sidewalks, parents fear for their children's safety, buses are always available, and once teens get their driver's license, forget about it.

Meanwhile, while Congress debates the appropriation of transportation funds for safer walking and bicycling options nationwide, New York City has created a Safe Routes to School program to facilitate pedestrian safety, and safer streets means more walking children. With $3 million in federal funds and a total budget of $5.5 million, the city has focused on traffic issues at 135 schools, about 10 percent of schools in the city's five boroughs.

In New York, the obesity problem is particularly severe. A 2003 survey of 3,000 children in kindergarten through fifth grade found 24 percent to be obese, up from 20 percent in a comparable survey taken seven years earlier. And about half the city's 1.1 million schoolkids were found to be overweight. That's hardly a surprise. In 2001, the City Council found that 41 percent of elementary schools and 23 percent of high schools did not provide regular PE classes; two years later, the council reported that 94 percent of all schools had no athletic fields. The council estimated that almost $1 billion was needed to upgrade and renovate facilities.

As a product of the city's system, I have seen the lack of facilities and legendary neglect. My high school in Brooklyn was constructed in 1960 with no running track or soccer field. The track team practiced in the basement hallway. I was reminded of that handicap when I saw the recent account of a New York City gym teacher in the South Bronx holding her class in the lobby of the building, constantly interrupted by students going to the bathroom and deliveries to the cafeteria. The teacher, like my coach, made do, but that's not good enough.

NEW YORK PROACTIVE IN STUDENT ACTIVITY

Private organizations have come to New York's rescue. The New York Road Runners, through its foundation, operates a number of school-centered running programs reaching tens of thousands of youngsters in New York and other cities. After a 1999 *New York Times* series detailing the decay in school sports facilities, Take the Field, a nonprofit group, was established to refurbish high school grounds. In its first five years, the organization raised $133 million and rebuilt facilities at forty-two high schools.

As a result of the obesity statistics of 2003, New York hired a public schools fitness and physical education director, Lori Rose

Benson. There are few more unwieldy bureaucracies than the New York City Board of Education. But Benson was given a team of ten regional directors, and by 2007 the city had a Kid Fitness for Schools program with a workout DVD and public television series in more than 9,700 elementary school classrooms.

What a breath of fresh air compared with old-style PE. Part cultural icon for its dumb-jock Hollywood portrayals, part social stigma for exposing bad bodies in bad outfits, and part permanent scarring for boot-camp-like tests such as rope climbing, the physical education class has been easy to dismiss as dopey and ineffectual. But with sweeping changes in the past decade moving it from skills-based goals to a fitness approach, PE is essential, especially given the six hours a day kids spend in front of the TV and computer screen.

But only one state, Illinois, has daily phys ed in all grades. Few states require elementary schools to have certified PE teachers. The latest figures for 2007 show that the nationwide average for required high school PE is one credit in four years.

In New Jersey, where I live, we're ranked second to Illinois in gym class requirements, according to newspaper reports. The state's PE statute—requiring 150 minutes a week of "blended" health and PE in all grades, apportioned by local school districts—dates back to 1917, when it was seen as a way to improve the physical fitness of recruits in World War I. There have been various political attempts to trim that requirement, but all failed under public pressure. "We've come full circle," James Mc-Call, Ph.D., coordinator of health and physical education for the state Department of Education, told me. "All the educational organizations are now supporting education of the whole child." Thank God, since among low-income children New Jersey has the highest incidence of childhood obesity of any state.

For schools, it seems easier to address food issues than physical activity because healthier eating has no effect on class schedules. When in 2004 Congress enacted the Child Nutrition and

Women, Infants and Children Reauthorization Act—ordering
schools participating in federally mandated school lunch and
breakfast programs to encourage physical activity and reduce fat-
tening foods in school lunches—many schools and some states
jumped on the nutrition idea. In Louisiana, for example, the Pennington Biomedical Research Center of Baton Rouge, in cooper-
ation with the state Department of Education, presented a list of
more than 200 food items that met healthy standards of calories,
fat, and sugar for school vending machines. As one expert put it,
hungry kids will eat just about anything, so why not carrots instead of fries?

However, many researchers, including BettyLou Sherry,
Ph.D., an epidemiologist at the CDC specializing in obesity, claim
that kids' poor diet is determined much more at home than in
school. Sherry told me that "portion size is out of control" and
that the megasize sodas that kids slurp are purchased primarily by
parents. Sherry also noted that her own studies have shown that
for cultural reasons black and Latino families had a greater acceptance of their children being overweight than white families
did. This finding mirrored the 2003 New York City elementary
school survey, which found 31 percent of Hispanic children and
23 percent of black children obese, as compared with 16 percent
and 14 percent for white and Asian youngsters, respectively.

Cultural differences aside, Steve Blair, Ph.D., professor of exercise science, epidemiology, and biostatistics at the University
of South Carolina, expressed skepticism of the headline-making
vending machine cutbacks, emphasizing the need for additional
research. "We're a society that likes simplistic solutions," said
Blair, previously president and CEO of the Cooper Institute in
Dallas. Blair said there are data showing that schoolchildren
make an average of 1.5 vending machine purchases per week,
and there was no way to know for sure, based on current research, whether eliminating those purchases would improve kids'
health (see interview, page 31).

THE GREAT CUPCAKE CRACKDOWN

More research might also settle a few scores in the great "cupcake crackdown" controversy. When parents at a school in our New Jersey district found out that bringing in nutritionally incorrect cupcakes for kids' birthdays was no longer permitted, they protested—and far more vigorously than over issues such as school funding. New Jersey is tame. To quote the *New York Times* in a 2007 school nutrition story: "Parents in Texas lobbied to get a 'Safe Cupcake Amendment' added to the state's nutrition policy. The measure, which passed, ensures that parents may bring frosted treats to schools for celebrations."

The cupcake dispute, while good for a laugh, reflects distorted parental values—"demand-free," as one psychiatrist put it on the *Today* show—and how our society compromises children's well-being. The latest rage in "active children" indulgence, at least in California, are kids and teen health clubs such as Fitwize4kids in Los Angeles and Overtime Fitness in the Silicon Valley. This burgeoning high-priced market for the MySpace generation comes with personal trainers for the kids, teens chatting on cell phones while sitting on exercise bikes, and, as one high school sophomore told the *New York Times*, a quick dash in the middle of a workout to buy a hot dog. In recognition of the mandate to avoid bruised egos, one trainer said, "You can't use the word 'wrong,' as in, 'You're doing the exercise wrong.'"

This "Generation Me" attitude, fueled by reality TV, obsession with celebrity, and the rise of social networking Web sites, stems in part, say some social scientists, from baby boom parents and educators who in the 1970s became fixated on instilling self-esteem in their children. We baby boomers get blamed for a lot. When we started the running movement in the 1970s, we were charged with narcissism, given our social activism of the 1960s. But the times they were a-changing. Our running may have had something to do with perfection of the self, but we shunned the spotlight, seeking a quiet, personal glory; if anything, running taught us humility.

Running also taught us about our bodies, but doctors did not always keep pace. I believe it was this void that led the American Academy of Pediatrics in 2003 to urge obesity screening with use of the new body mass index, or BMI, a rough measure of body fat, that is a kind of Cliffs Notes for physicians.

BMI is a doctor tool, not a patient tool. BMI is almost impossible for the average person to calculate, but you can go to various Web sites such as the CDC's, enter a child's height, weight, age, and gender, obtain the magic number, and see if it's within healthy levels. Your doctor can tell you if, say, a child is in the 95th percentile, signifying obesity. (However, Betty Sherry, the CDC obesity expert, told me that "'overweight' was the terminology more accepted for children—although that's being debated— to help avoid the stigma" of the term "obesity.")

In any case, what happened to simple height and weight? "BMI," said Sherry, "is a little better than weight-for-height measurement in assessing body fat. Doctors have to translate this for parents into meaningful language." Sherry added, "BMI is a screening tool. We need to emphasize the role of the family. You don't want kids to lose weight. You want them to grow into their height."

With such ambiguity, it was not surprising to learn from a *New York Times* article titled "America's Epidemic of Youth Obesity" that the National Institutes of Health was financing "no fewer than 16 studies" to find ways to encourage a healthier lifestyle for young people. The time it takes for families to prepare healthy meals was said to be a major stumbling block.

BETTER MEALS ARE EASIER THAN YOU THINK

But as best-selling author Michael Pollan (*In Defense of Food*) said in a television interview, healthy food preparation is easier and less time-consuming than most people think. He blamed food network celebrity chefs and their fussy dishes for creating a chic but labor-intensive aura around food when all it takes is a little garlic and olive oil to get a good meal going.

But how do we stop the fast-food juggernaut when there's a McDonald's even in the lobby of the Hospital of the University of Pennsylvania in Philadelphia? I've seen it. People mill around outside clutching their Happy Meals. The hospital handbook, referring to patients, states, "Your child may order food from McDonald's once a week unless indicated in the diet order by the doctor or physician." Who knew that health-conscious patients, shunning the Quarter Pounder, would ever make hospital food their first choice?

An inactive youngster does not need a supersized diet to become obese. Researchers say that a small energy imbalance (little activity and just a little more food) can tip the scales. An extra soft drink per day, 150 calories, will result in a 15-pound weight gain in a year. In a few years, that's 50 pounds.

If only an extra Coke was all we had to worry about. The food industry spends around $10 billion a year marketing to children— much of it, according to Senator Tom Harkin of Iowa, promoting sugary and nutritionally poor products. Harkin, a longtime advocate of initiatives to stem childhood obesity, has sought to legislate restrictions on advertising to children. In 2005, Kraft Foods announced it would halt television advertising of certain products it considered unhealthy to children under 12.

Needless to say, food lobbyists have objected to Harkin's efforts, pointing to research showing that lack of exercise is the real problem. Others in favor of industry change said such claims were being used as a distraction from the unhealthy food products marketed to kids.

AN EXPERT FOCUSES ON CALORIC BALANCE

Is it too much food, too little activity, or both? Steve Blair takes a contrary view of childhood obesity, or what he terms "positive caloric balance." He says that too much emphasis has been given to the food intake part of the equation and that up to now there have been no concrete data showing children are indeed eating more than they used to. Maybe they are, said Blair, but more studies are needed to find out. At the same time, he said, his instinct was that the problem rested more with lack of activity, or energy expenditure. To obtain answers, he and colleagues had a major federally funded study in the works. Blair said the scope of the childhood obesity problem required no less than a "Manhattan Project" approach.

I believe that we can start to have an impact by helping a few kids—or a few hundred—here and there, with innovative, constructive ideas, but more than that we need to respect children and appreciate that, given half a chance, they will do the right thing. Kids *want* to be active. They *want* to eat good foods. They *want* to feel good.

Our greatest offense as adults has been allowing the worst of our many unhealthy sins to pass on to our children—and thinking that it's okay. We'd all benefit from more efforts like the Edible Schoolyard in Berkeley, California, organized by health food pioneer Alice Waters. Started in 1996, Edible Schoolyard is a public schools gardening and cooking project in which students prepare their own fresh food for lunch, and food-related activities are woven into the curriculum. As Waters described in a 2006 *New York Times* op-ed article, "We're not scaring them [children] with the health consequences of their eating habits;

we're engaging them in interactive education that brings them into a new relationship with food. Nothing less will change their behavior."

If we give kids some responsibility, dramatic change can occur. It's nice to see million-dollar running tracks, but take kids out to any field or park and with a little motivation they will run their legs off. As with exercise, kids enjoy food preparation and will take pride in what they create. Preparing a meal requires care, tenderness, and a kind of love, especially when done with loved ones. "We need a revolution, a delicious revolution," Waters wrote. "I know from experience that teaching children about food changes their lives."

Let's all work for changes in kids' lives. We already have a kids' running revolution gathering steam. Let's help running capture every child possible, every teenager, every family, school and community, and start to bring about lasting improvement in kids' health and well-being.

▶ Steve Blair on Childhood Obesity

Steven N. Blair, Ph.D., is a former president and CEO of Cooper Institute in Dallas and currently a professor of exercise science, epidemiology, and biostatistics at the University of South Carolina. Blair, one of the nation's preeminent health scientists, spent twenty-two years at Cooper, from 1984 to 2006, working on fitness and exercise. At USC, he is embarking on what may be the most important study yet of childhood obesity. The federally funded project involves several leading institutions nationwide.

Q: Are you optimistic that we can turn this problem around anytime soon?
Blair: Clearly, we're in the midst of a worldwide childhood obesity epidemic. It's been going on for twenty-five years. It involves

nearly every country and age group. Where I depart from a lot of other people is, I don't think we know the cause. The fundamental thermodynamic reason is: positive caloric balance.

Then, to take the next step, what's causing this? Is it that people are eating more calories than they used to, or are they expending fewer calories, or could it be a combination of the two? When pinned down, most people will say it's a combination. If you did a search of the popular press, the amount of space devoted to the intake [food] side of the equation would dwarf the amount devoted to the expenditure [activity] side. Most of the strategies that have been touted, like restricting sugary drinks and getting vending machines out of schools, are related to intake.

Q: Aren't those good ideas?
Blair: We have no compelling evidence that the average daily caloric intake in the United States has gone up over the period of the obesity epidemic. You can find bits and pieces [of evidence] here and there, but we have never seen fit to try and get good estimates of average daily caloric expenditure. So we don't know.

Q: But we do know that youngsters have been getting less and less exercise, don't we?
Blair: It's not whether kids have reported more or less physical activity on surveys. That's not the question. The question is, what's happened to energy expenditure? It's energy expenditure and energy intake that determine caloric balance.

Q: Surely we know what we see around us.
Blair: In every aspect of life we have engineered energy expenditure down. But we don't have any real data. It's a gut feel.

Q: Can't we trust our gut?
Blair: It may be reliable, but it's not data. In the absence of data, I submit that we do not know.

Q: If the educated guesses are done by reputable people, and we do things like removing school vending machines and changing school lunches while increasing physical activity, aren't those good ideas?

Blair: Possibly, maybe even probably. But since we don't know the specific causes, how in the world can we come up with rational strategies? Dig a little deeper into the vending machine issue: take any school district, and the data show that the average number of purchases per week is 1.5. Is eliminating that amount of calories enough to have a major effect? We do not know.

Q: Most of the response to obesity has focused on diet?

Blair: In the case of diet, and more so with adults than kids, we have spent tens of millions of dollars in dietary and nutrition surveys. And I still stand by my statement: There's no compelling evidence that average daily caloric intake has gone up. We're putting too much emphasis on diet.

Q: There should be more emphasis in the expenditure area.

Blair: That's my bias, but there's no data there either. It's a quandary.

Q: How do we obtain the necessary information?

Blair: At the university, we're trying to mount a study that will get better answers to these questions. One of our projects is called an age overlapping cohort study. We're going to recruit large numbers of kids, ages 6, 9, 12, and 15, and follow each age group for three to four years. My colleague Russ Pate is leader of the study. I co-chair the energy balance committee. We're working with other universities. We hope to get better data on energy expenditure. Otherwise we're foundering in the dark.

Q: But we can't wait for those results to take action.

Blair: No. In general, I would promote healthy eating and regular physical activity. An Institute of Medicine report on childhood obesity that came out a few years ago listed at least fifteen strategies, and they emphasized that you could not cherry-pick, you had to be doing all of it. That includes public policy, community, schools, medical . . .

Q: We need a national movement in all these areas.
Blair: We don't put our money where our mouth is. As a society, we jump all over this as a huge problem, but the vast majority of what comes out of it is lip service. If it's as big a problem as the federal government says, then it calls for a "Manhattan Project" level of commitment.

Q: Why do you think our society is lagging here?
Blair: Going back to vending machines, we're a society that likes simple solutions, a magic bullet. H. L. Mencken said a century ago: "For every complex problem, there's a simple solution that does not work."

Q: Considering your self-confessed energy expenditure bias, I imagine you'd advocate running for children.
Blair: Running, but not only running. We have data showing that if kids are outside, they burn more calories than if they're inside. Get them out. Encourage activity. I applaud the efforts of the running community.

Q: Who are your partners in your study?
Blair: We are working with the University of Iowa, Cooper Institute, Winthrop University in South Carolina, and Pennington Biomedical Research Center in Baton Rouge. We will have samples of kids from each area. We want to obtain good data to help community activists, to help us sharpen our focus for better strategies. The next wave of studies can use that information and develop interventions.

Q: What's the timetable?

Blair: Phase one is a congressional earmark through the Department of Defense. We sold it to the politicians on that basis. The name is Troop Recruit Improvement Methods (TRIM). Where's the fighting force going to come from? Now we're trying to get phase two going, the money.

2

Running with Smiles

I try to make it loosey-goosey. I want to hook kids on running. I want to put that sparkle in their eye. I want all smiles.

—BILL SUMNER, COACH AND KIDS' RUNNING
PROGRAM DIRECTOR IN CALIFORNIA

Not long ago at a Jewish Community Center in a New York City suburb, I attended the ceremonial Hebrew naming of a newborn. Lunch was served after the ritual prayers and song, and the twenty or so young children in attendance sat with rare reticence as they picked at their meal. We adults marveled at their behavior.

But as soon as lunch was over, the whole bunch of them, ages 3 to 7, started running in spontaneous fashion all over the room, about the size of a small gym. Some ran in circles. Some darted across the room, scooting around adults trying to prevent their coffee from spilling. Some ran in a line, one behind the other, as though in a camp game.

They would not stop. The kids found inventive ways to duck around chairs and tables and people, keeping up the pace while eluding the outstretched arms of nervous moms and dads. What the children had in common was unbridled energy, excitement, big smiles, and laughter.

These youngsters were expressing their natural urge to move and play. It's an urge seen all the time in children, whether they're running down the street, chasing a squirrel in the backyard, or, increasingly participating in kids' races and running programs found around the country. Watch children on the run. They fly: arms jutting out, knees high, feet kicking back, heads up. No rules, just pure joy. It is a joy, I would suggest, that gets to the heart of human existence—a joy that touched the great medical man and running philosopher George Sheehan, who above all else implored adults to reach back into their inner child and "play."

That joyful spirit is reflected in the style of coaches such as Bill Sumner, a kind of running Pied Piper from southern California who directs the kids' Introduction to Running program affiliated with the Orange County Marathon. The youngsters run 2.5 miles a week for ten weeks, then do 1.2 miles on the day of the marathon to complete their own "marathon," 26.2 miles total. "Kids run carefree, with a smile on their faces," says Sumner. "It's hard to find a kid who's grunting and grinding. If you do find one, you calm him down. I try to make it loosey-goosey. I want to hook kids on running. I want to put that sparkle in their eye. I want all smiles."

PLAY PROVIDES FREEDOM

Three words come up repeatedly when I speak with experts on children and running: "smiles," "play," and "fun." Make running a form of play and kids will smile. Make it a serious business and in due time they probably won't. "Play refers to the young child's activities characterized by freedom from all but personally imposed rules . . . and by the absence of any goals outside of the activity itself," the noted child psychologist Bruno Bettelheim once wrote. In the same essay, in the *Atlantic Monthly*, Bettelheim referred to the philosopher John Locke's view that recreation must include "delight" and that when children experience the diversion of play they must be permitted to do it "after their own fashion."

If the kids running around the community center that day were stopped by adults and organized into some structured running with rules that limited spontaneity, you can bet they would have objected or just quit. Play would have ended and smiles and laughter would have disappeared.

In our maddening, nonstop techno-culture, overscheduled, test-taking kids are at the breaking point. It is hard to imagine a better endeavor for constructive, pressure-free play than running—as long as the running is "miles of smiles." But running for children is too often undermined by parents and coaches dishing out adult-style mandates and performance requirements, and then it becomes one more burdensome hurdle on a child's after-school list.

People of my generation are said to drift into gooey nostalgia when recalling the purity of our made-up games and choose-up-sides street play. Guilty as charged. In my Brooklyn neighborhood, we played ball and held races till we dropped, gaining a wealth of benefits that no one ever preached were good for us but which were propelled by the inexhaustible urge to have fun. Our block was a laboratory. We learned about risks and boundaries, sharing and sportsmanship, and which sports we liked best. We also learned the give-and-take of negotiation and to appreciate hard work, and we gained some humility by making the most of small, urban spaces. There were no lush, green parks in my 'hood.

FUN TOPS KIDS' DESIRES

Our Brooklyn-style passion for sports play would have been consistent with the findings of a 1990 landmark study of 10,000 children ages 10 to 18 by researchers Martha Ewing and Vern Seefeldt of Michigan State University. Asked their motives for participation, boys' top five responses were (1) to have fun, (2) to improve skills, (3) for the excitement of competition, (4) to do something they're good at, and (5) to stay in shape. Girls' top five were (1) to have fun, (2) to stay in shape, (3) to get exercise, (4) to improve skills, and (5) to do something they're good at. "To win" was number eight for boys and twelfth and last for girls.

It should be no surprise to see fun topping both lists. Do we even know what fun is anymore? We call many kids' races "fun runs" to distinguish them from supposedly hard-nosed competitions. Shouldn't the term "fun run" be redundant? Shouldn't *every* run, especially for children, be fun? Are "fun" and "fast" mutually exclusive?

I think we're a little mixed up here. It's not so much the pace and intent of a run that might detract from the fun, but the entire context in which children are running from day to day and week to week. A child taught to enjoy running as play can have loads of fun even while seeking personal bests; another child, taught the wrong lessons from the start, can feel dissatisfied even while jogging.

A BEAUTIFUL FRIENDSHIP

Look at it this way: Kids need and want play. Kids need and want running. This must be the start of a beautiful friendship.

A February 2008 *New York Times Magazine* cover story, "Taking Play Seriously," by Robin Marantz Henig, rings so true. She leads off with psychiatrist Stuart Brown, president of the National Institute for Play, speaking rhapsodically about play as essential to children and adults and emphasizing the long-term consequences of play deprivation. Henig quotes Brown telling a sold-out New York Public Library audience of concerned parents: "If you look at what produces learning and memory and well-being, play is as fundamental as any other aspect of life, including sleep and dreams."

As the article states, play takes many forms. A 6-year-old enjoys running as play in different ways than a 16-year-old. But regardless of age, play is a "behavioral kaleidoscope," a repertory, according to Mark Bekoff, an evolutionary biologist at the University of Colorado, also quoted by Henig. What I take most from her many scientific points, as applied to running, is that play gives children choices, control, and responsibility—indeed, a responsibility to learn based on a menu of opportunity. Children learn innovation and creativity. And at a time when so much information is merely a click away, running offers the thrill of discovery.

Play is, ultimately, about freedom. Running, too, is about freedom. Running and play together have the power to change children, families, schools, communities. "Look at life without play, and it's not much of a life," Stuart Brown is quoted at the end of the *Times* story. "If you think of all the things we do that are play-related and erase those, it's pretty hard to keep going."

It's clear that running must be kept as play, that adults see the light and let kids be kids, as they move their bodies, on trails and tracks, in gyms and parks—smiling all the way—and even, as the case may be, at a reception hall where prayers are spoken and songs are sung. Let's find out more about getting kids running for fun, fitness, and long-lasting health and well-being.

EARLY INTERVENTION

The effects of very early activity can pave the way for physical expression later on, according to Daniel Gould, Ph.D., a sports psychologist at Michigan State and director of the school's Institute for Study of Youth Sports. He likens it to children who read better if parents read to them when they're young. Before kids can even walk, engage them in play on the floor, suggests Gould. Dance with your child. Use physical activity toys. Buy plenty of balls. When the child reaches toddler age, play chasing games in the backyard. Get kids jumping, running, hopping, and throwing, says Gould.

TODDLER TROTS

While age 3 or 4 is too young for any real running—kids' bodies are not developed enough and they don't have the attention span—they can still participate in the Toddler Trots or Diaper Dashes of up to 100 yards that are sprouting up at family-oriented running events. Just point them in the right direction, get your cameras ready . . . and watch them go! Children will start learning good habits and pick up family cues that running is something to do and has rewards, whether a medal, hug, or ice pop. "As long as the child is capable of running without falling down, it's okay to run in brief spurts," says Dr. Teri McCambridge, a Baltimore pediatrician who chairs the American Academy of Pediatrics Sports Medicine and Fitness Committee. Don't let a 3- or 4-year-old run loose without supervision because their vision is not yet mature, making it difficult for them to track and judge the speed of moving objects.

FIRST STRIDES

At school age, 5 or 6, kids are developed enough, physically, emotionally, and intellectually, to get into the practice of running. They have some ability to focus and a short but adequate attention span—enough to follow basic instructions and function in a group. They learn by trial and error and need "space" for learning. Have them join with other children in running. Play tag games. Have kids run around cones, flags, soccer balls, or stuffed animals. They should run in short bursts. They'll go fast, peter out, then want to sprint again. Have them run like animals with movements of rabbits, horses, or butterflies. Set kids up in relays in which they slap another child's hand as a "pass." Have kids run through hoops or from tree to tree.

In his City Sports for Kids track program, under the auspices of the New York Road Runners Foundation, head coach Bob Glover (co-author of the best-selling *Competitive Runner's Handbook*) has the youngest kids play Road Runner, in which they run a couple of laps of a 200-meter track, then hide behind a coach. Or the children will run a lap or two, then sit down for a running-related story like one in the Berenstain Bears series.

If children tire and want to stop, let them. Walking is fine too. Just don't let kids get bored. Don't have them run in a straight line for long. When I ran years ago with my young daughters, at corners I would put out my hand to indicate left or right turn. They pleaded embarrassment, but I think they liked the bit. I also sang songs and played games in which I asked them to guess what I was describing, which could be a friend, a fruit, or anything in between.

Think outside the box. The Big Sur Marathon's Just Run kids' program in California has a "principals' challenge," in which school kids chase the principal around a track or field. "The principal gets a 50-yard head start," says program founder Mike Dove. He's learned that when you send kids around a path for a certain number of laps, instead of just calling out, "Lap three . . . two to go," tell them they will get a hand stamp after each lap with an animal or star on it. It's a great motivator and source of pride. "Kids go home and tell their parents, 'Look, I got five stamps on my hand,'" says Dove.

Dove, 61, a top masters runner, has learned other devices in nurturing the youngest athletes. When kids run relays on a loop around a soccer ball 40 yards downfield, he finds that about 80 percent of them will run around the ball from the right side. He has the children alternate right and left to promote agility and balance and to strengthen different muscle groups. And the kids enjoy changing directions.

PUNISHMENT TABOO

Never use running as a form of punishment, not even in the most subtle, implicit way. No extra laps or whatever for a child not paying attention or some other misdeed. Have your radar set for your child's soccer or basketball practice, where coaches tend to dish out such nonsense. If necessary, be ready to convert a negative into a positive by reinforcing all the happy talk your running child should already know.

DRESS FOR SUCCESS

Kids are fussy about what they run in, especially as they get older, and should not be held to adult standards of running attire. They can run in extra-long shorts and goofy shirts; they don't always need the "right" fabrics and styling. Encourage kid-pleasing get-ups, even costumes, if that helps get them out the door. Unless it's hot, don't fret over something heavy tiring them out. There's a children's run in East Lansing, Michigan, the Dinosaur Dash 5K, in which the kids run or walk in dinosaur headdresses. A Bronto-saurus Blitz 3K youth race in Tustin, California, drew 2,458 par-ticipants in 2008, making it the third largest children's event in the state. You can't go wrong with kids and dinosaurs.

PUSH, PULL, PROD

Experts say not to push kids to run but instead let them decide, let them ask—but is that always the best strategy? There are many things that children like and need but don't jump at; they can often do with a little prodding. Some kids are shy and may not welcome the idea of joining other kids in running. But run-ning is also a way to break that shyness and make new friends, a huge incentive. As Deena Kastor, the 2004 Olympic marathon bronze medalist, once told me, "I was a painfully shy child; that's why my parents pushed me into running. It made all the differ-ence with socialization and self-esteem. For me, running meant going to practice to be with friends."

Find a middle ground between taking your lead from the child and prodding, says Gould, the Michigan sports psychologist. He cautions adults not to let prodding become an excuse to push kids too far. In his studies on what he calls the "professionalism of youth sports," Gould has found large numbers of "overin-volved" parents interfering with their child's development as an athlete or person.

BEST PLACES TO RUN

While it's usually easiest to run from the front door, paved roads are hard on children's legs, and sidewalks and traffic limit options for fun and games. Still, for time-pressured parents, there's noth-ing wrong with taking young ones around the block a few times.

Dr. Bill Roberts, past president of the American College of Sports Medicine and medical director of the Twin Cities Marathon, measured a quarter mile from his house and had his kids at 5 and 6 (after they asked) run out and back, a half mile, a few times a week. When kids are older, you can run the roads as transportation, to an ice cream parlor or, in the case of Albuquerque coach Adam Kedge, to a bagel shop for Sunday brunch. Kedge and his sons, 8 and 9, do a 2-mile "bagel run," eat, then run 2 miles back, all the while calling themselves by the names of local running stars.

But out on the roads, there's always risk that parents running with children will "carry" them too far, beyond their enjoyment and what's good for them. Most 7-, 8-, or 9-year-olds should not be doing an adult-level 5 or 6 miles at a clip.

Try going to parks, fields, and tracks. At parks, grass surfaces, dirt trails, and wooded paths are great for varied loops and distances, seeing other people, animals and wildlife, getting shade from the sun, finding water fountains and bathrooms, creating imaginative running games, and running hills, which kids love. Pushing up is a challenge (and teaches kids to coordinate arms and legs); flying down is a game. Soccer and ball fields are simple but serviceable. Kids can do laps, cut across, stop and sprint, run the bases; a little open space goes a long way.

Tracks offer precise distances, and running laps does not have to be tedious, as some say. They're ideal for relays, for alternating walking and running, for motivating kids with distance goals like running a mile and hitting certain times. Always vary the distance, and use time goals sparingly. Most tracks circle a football or soccer field, so you have a grassy area for more variation. It's easy to reward laps covered with ribbons, stickers, bookmarks, and such, or use the Just Run hand-stamp idea.

One school in the Just Run program, Carmel River Elementary, has a two-lane, 200-meter track that kids use during PE class and recess. It's easy to keep records of laps run and distance covered and integrate all the calculations into classroom teaching, says the principal, Jay Marden, a former national-caliber 10,000-meter runner.

In New York City, Public School 102 in East Harlem, part of the New York Road Runners Foundation Mighty Milers program, benefits from having a track a block away. PE teacher Steve Sloan takes students from pre-K through fifth grade to the track for laps. Each student runs a mile or more at least twice a week (some walk). In the 2007–8 term, the youngsters averaged over 200 miles per student for the school term. He says, "One day a fourth grader told me, 'This is getting easier every time I do it.' I told him, 'That's what I've been waiting to hear.'" Sloan says he has some youngsters up to 10 laps, more than 2 miles.

While tracks can inspire children to improve, they can also call attention to the slowest kids, who need to know that there are many measures of success, not just a lap count or time.

When Dr. Jennifer Sluder, a pediatrician at Childrens Hospital Los Angeles, observed schoolchildren running on a track for a research project, she found one excited boy who came up to her and said, "Last time I finished last. This time I wasn't. I've been running with my grandmother two times a week."

"HOT LEMON PIE"

From first to last, children need to feel proud about their running, and oftentimes they take their cues from adults. Steve Sloan gives his kids nicknames like "Sofast," "Hot Lemon Pie," and "Ice Cream Sandwich" as a caring identity that, he says, builds character and positive thinking. "If I call you 'Sofast,' it means you have to live up to it," he says. California coach Bill Sumner meets and greets every youngster in his large group with a jibe of recognition. "Kids want fitness, but more than that, they want attention," he says. "They want me knowing their names, saying hello."

When giving youngsters feedback, parents should be aware of body language, tone of voice, gestures. "Kids have antennae. They can pick up whether you really mean it," says Philadelphia sports psychologist Joel Fish, Ph.D., author, with Susan Magee, of *101 Ways to Be a Terrific Sports Parent*. Kids are keen enough, says Fish, to tell when a parent says he's proud of a child's running effort but comes across as being disappointed.

STRETCH IT OUT

As soon as they start to run, kids can also begin stretching exercises. They benefit not only from limbering up but also from developing routines and discipline and, in a group, working with others to foster a team atmosphere. Dr. Brenda Armstrong, a pediatric cardiologist and coach with the Durham Striders youth team in North Carolina, says that kids as young as 5 can understand group protocol. Her squad does stretching exercises to a count of 10 or 20, which builds on attention span and focuses children for the rest of the practice session. At 6, children begin to improve posture and balance, important qualities in handling various stretches (see below for a complete stretching program).

▶ Stretching Exercises for Children

Awarding-winning PE teacher and marathoner Pat Mantone of Marlboro, New Jersey, advocates this stretching routine for young runners of all ages. These exercises, says Mantone, will stimulate blood flow to the working muscles, and loosen and strengthen muscles to help prevent injury. She has her students, and run-

ners she works with, stretch before and after running. Before
running, they do the entire routine; after running, they do a few
of the more gentle stretches, avoiding any jumping movements.
Mantone generally holds stretches for a count of 20. She finds
kids enjoy counting, which helps their focus and attention span.
She emphasizes that stretches should be done gently, with no
fast, jerking motions. (For additional stretches, see chapter 5,
page 107.)

1. Seated bend. In a seated position, bend legs and put feet
together in front of body so the soles touch, and lean forward from the waist while grasping your toes. Bring your
nose toward your feet. As you count, try to go lower and
lower, feeling muscles stretching. Most kids won't get their
nose all the way down at first. (Older kids can put elbows
on knees, pressing knees to the ground.) *Benefits:* thigh
muscles and lower back.

2. Hurdlers' stretch. In seated position with the sole of one
foot on the thigh of the other foot, reach with both hands to
your toes, bringing your nose toward the knee. Do both
sides. *Benefits:* hamstring muscles and lower back.

3. Leg reach. In seated position, extend legs in front of you
and reach for the feet, trying to touch your heels. *Benefits:*
hamstring muscles, gluteals (rear), calves, and lower back.

4. Squat reach. Stand in squatting position with left leg forward and bent, knee to chest, and right leg extended back
with heel flush on ground. Reach with right hand to right
foot. Do both sides. *Benefits:* Achilles tendons, upper legs,
and plantar fascia (band in feet).

5. Sit-ups. Lying on your back with legs bent, knees up, and
hands across chest, lift the torso up and forward as far as
you can toward your knees. (Those having difficulty can
grab a pant leg for leverage.) Do 10 to 50 depending on age.
Benefits: abdominal muscles and lower back.

6. Push-ups. Assume push-up position with arms shoulder width apart, body raised, and feet extended back. (Those having difficulty can do modified push-ups, resting knees on floor.) Do 10 to 20 depending on age. *Benefits:* arms, shoulders, and abs.

7. Coffee grinder. From standing position, lower body, place one hand on the ground, and spin around in a circle, feeling pressure on your arm. Do both sides 10 times each. *Benefits:* arms.

8. Mountain climb. Get into a sprinter's crouch with hands flat on the ground shoulder width apart, and alternate bringing your feet back and forth from rear to arms. Do up to 50. *Benefits:* gluteal muscles (the "power" muscles in running).

9. Standing jumps. Find a line, bend knees, feel your weight in your lower legs and feet, and jump forward and back, then side to side. Do 20 to 40 each movement. *Benefits:* lower leg and gluteal strength plus balance and coordination. (Older kids can also do the same with hopping.)

10. Jumping jacks. Do 20, touching hands above heads. Groups should do them in unison, counting together. *Benefits:* full body conditioning.

WHEN KIDS FEEL PAIN

Children face little risk of injury from running as long as they are not pushed too hard, or, as Dr. Bill Roberts says, they don't do "too much, too soon, too hard, too often." Kids tend to have more sense than adults when it comes to gauging fatigue. As Mike Dove of California's Just Run program notes, "When a 5-year-old gets tired, he just stops." Kids listen to pain, says Dr. Teri McCambridge. "I don't think many kids would choose to run through pain."

Dan Gould, the sports psychologist, says youngsters should

learn the difference between routine discomfort from training, like stiff muscles, and pain that signifies injury. Coaches, he says, should discuss this, even with young children. The first sign of an injury, other than a child's complaint, may be a change in gait, says Dr. McCambridge. Check to see whether the child is striding normally or limping. She says that kids who do experience pain will usually be affected in the growth centers, which develop at different stages in a sequential pattern from the feet up. Typically, a 9-year-old would have heel pain, an 11-year-old would have knee pain, and a 13-year-old would have hip pain.

Some kids will run through pain, to try to show toughness or not to let teammates down; sometimes they even do it with the consent of a parent or coach. Every doctor's rule, as expressed by Dr. Deborah Squires, chief of pediatric sports medicine at Duke University Medical Center, is: "If a child says he's hurt or tired, he must be allowed to stop." And the child should not be given anti-inflammatory medication such as Advil (ibuprofen) in order to run, says Dr. McCambridge, because developing bone could be seriously damaged if the pain signals are suppressed.

Unfortunately, there's no way to know how much force the growing skeleton can tolerate, says Dr. Stephen G. Rice, director of the Jersey Shore Sports Medicine Center at Jersey Shore University Medical Center in Neptune, New Jersey, and a specialist in children's sports. Dr. Rice says that children need to feel that they can regulate their activity and have an acceptable "exit strategy" if a run or workout proves too difficult.

A common discomfort that few youngsters avoid is the benign but painful side stitch, which is still not fully understood. It may occur from eating too soon before running or a runner's breathing pattern. One tip to eliminate a stitch on a run comes from Don Kardong, a 1976 Olympic marathoner, who states in the Road Runners Club of America "Children's Running Guide for Teachers and Coaches": "Pretend your stomach is a balloon, filling with air when you inhale, deflating when you exhale. The air is really going into your lungs, not your stomach, but this trick seems to work. It may help to massage the stitch at the same time."

DISTANCE AND AGE

Most running programs and health professionals advise modest distances of a quarter mile or half mile for kids of 5 or 6 or a little older, with gradual increases depending on interest and aptitude as they age. For example, the Fit for Life Kids Challenge in the Richmond, Virginia, area, for kids starting at 5, recommends walking or running at least a mile every other day for ten weeks, culminating with a mile fun run held on the same day as an adult 10K. At Carmel River Elementary in California, kindergarten kids start off with a quarter mile a day, while the oldest students, in fourth and fifth grades (ages 10–11), do as much as a mile a day. The national Girls on the Run program has its younger participants, in third through fifth grades, do a couple of miles twice a week.

Using time rather than distance, children of 7 or 8 could work up to 15 to 20 minutes of running (around 2 miles max) three times a week, which is about all their attention spans can manage. Dr. Rice says that youngsters 9 to 12 can increase to 30 to 45 minutes (3 to 4 miles) four to five times a week. But he cautions that because children have a shorter stride length than adults and therefore take more strides per mile, their musculoskeletal system absorbs more pounding. Fortunately, according to Dr. Armstrong, hard-running kids will usually run out of gas— "hitting the wall," as she puts it—before incurring an injury.

Still, as an added precaution, a parent who wants to take a youngster for a 4-mile run should first do 1 mile out and back and then, if the child feels okay, proceed with the last 2 miles, suggests Dr. Rice. That way, he adds, you won't risk getting a child in over his head.

Dr. Roberts agrees with these age/time suggestions but notes it's "hard to say whether a 9- or 10-year-old should do this or that. If kids enjoy running and don't get hurt, I would let them go as far as they want." In an extreme example of youth prowess and desire, one 10-year-old boy pleaded with his father to let him run the Twin Cities Marathon. The father resisted until the boy showed his mettle by running 56 laps around the block, totaling 26 miles. The boy ran the marathon, in about four hours, and when he was checked in the medical tent afterward, "he looked better than most adults," says Dr. Roberts. (That's a story to tell, not a practice to emulate.)

There's never been a study to determine safe, healthy mileage for a child's age, and much of what is known is based on trial and error. Dr. Armstrong and her colleagues at Duke University Medical Center believe that children's health, fitness, and competitive needs can be met safely by emphasizing short distances, speed work, and plenty of rest, which the Durham track squad lives by. The coaches do not let kids 10 and under race distances above 1,500 meters or a mile, and twice-weekly practices revolve around fast laps of the track with ample rest in between plus easy warm-up jogging. "We're always looking at the long term," she says.

To ensure long-lasting interest and well-being, children should not specialize in running year-round but rather should play a variety of sports. The more a child does other sports, the better off he'll be, says Dr. Rice, who notes, "Even while doing another sport, a youngster can still go out and run once a week."

YOUNG RACERS

Good feelings about running can be enhanced by competition. It's true that every race has only one winner, and parents tell me that children groomed into today's slam-dunk sports climate tend to feel that winning is everything and that even second place is a disappointment. Kids need to learn that there are many measures of personal success. Just showing up and participating is something to be proud of. Other measures of pride, according to sports psychologist Joel Fish, include giving your best effort, being a good teammate, learning something to make you a better runner, handling hilly terrain, helping another runner, and of course having fun. "Parents plant the important seeds," says Fish. "Don't put all the success eggs in one basket."

Kids should focus not on beating others but on self-improvement, says the sports psychologist Daniel Gould. "They should be judged on their own standards." Gould feels that cross-country offers ideal competition for youngsters since the team scoring system enables finishers back in the field to count as much as kids up front. Relays are also excellent for promoting teamwork and spreading the recognition around. But some kids, says Gould, worry about letting relay mates down with a poor performance. A fearful youngster should not be put on the anchor leg.

There's a welcome trend in youth races to do away with time and place and avoid performance pressures. The Peachtree Junior 3,000-meter event in Atlanta, for kids 7 to 12, is billed as "noncompetitive," with no results or awards. The field is limited to 2,500 and held in a park to enhance supervision. It's set up with races for each age—one for 7-year-olds, one for 8-year-olds, and so on—to promote camaraderie and fairness. In New Jersey, the Spring Lake 5-mile run, which has 7,000 adults on a Saturday morning, runs a dozen kids' races on Friday night, from 25 yards to a quarter mile, with over 1,900 participants ages 4 to 14. It's also billed as "noncompetitive," with no awards. Every finisher receives a medal, and all kids who preregister are guaranteed a T-shirt.

A 4-year-old may seem too young for racing, but 25 yards is just a quick little burst. In New York, youth coach Bob Glover has his City Sports kids start racing at 5 and 6 with "peewee"

runs of two blocks. They have a chant: "Start slow, finish fast."
Children like to take off at full speed. They need to learn pacing,
but you don't want to blunt their spontaneity either.

REWARD SYSTEM

Coaches and youth program coordinators say that incentives
such as T-shirts, certificates, or other trinkets help motivate kids
and give them a sense of identity, but some feel that external rewards condition children to feel they run only for a prize, not for
the intrinsic value. Some people have found a way to balance the
thrill of getting goodies with the thrill of a healthy run.

At Carmel River Elementary in California, students receive
foot tokens and lap markers for every 50 laps run on the school
track, which they wear on shoelaces or as a necklace, a testament to their miles. They also combine running with good deeds,
receiving coupons to redeem at the school store. New York's
Mighty Milers program showers student runners with T-shirts,
medals, water bottles, and pens. But the East Harlem teacher
Steve Sloan says he may start to cut back on incentives for his
345 children so "they don't run for a T-shirt or medal but because
it's good for you."

Sometimes, the extras can be more important to parents than
to their children. In New York, when Bob Glover saw parents
bringing their kids to Central Park races every weekend to col-
lect age-group trophies, he passed a New York Road Runners
rule that kids had to be at least 12 to win an award at a club-
sponsored event.

An event on Boston Marathon weekend seems to have come
up with the best solution yet, or at least one that is politically
correct. At the Heartbreak Hill International Youth race for
youngsters 9 and older—up and down the famous ascent for a

mile—every participant receives a seedling tree as a gift. The race has been going on for sixteen years and, says director Linda Plaut, "we have planted a forest around the world."

▶ Sneakers or Running Shoes: The Bare Facts

Do children need regulation running shoes when they start out running, even though they may be running only short distances a few times a week? Most experts say that authentic shoes are a must for proper support and injury prevention (not to mention comfort and speed), while anecdotal evidence suggests that some kids at least can enjoy running in basic sneakers.

Most of the youngsters I've seen in the Freehold Area Running Club kids' summer races in New Jersey (see chapter 3) compete in generic sneakers. Likewise, at Lynbrook Elementary in Springfield, Virginia, a Healthy School award winner, I saw mostly tennis and basketball-style sneakers on kids running the Pacer test in PE class (see chapter 4). While there's no data on whether an 8-year-old running in sneakers will have later injuries, the kids I saw seemed to experience no less pleasure, and were not any slower, than those with authentic running shoes.

Kids' running shoes cost about $40 to $60. Since kids can quickly outgrow shoes, parents (especially those with more than one child running) face a significant expense. In California, the Big Sur Marathon's Just Run program provides a limited number of shoes to low-income families. Just Run has been assisted by a local charitable group called HELP (Healthy Eating and Lifestyle Principles), which conducts a number of children's health initiatives in the area.

Just Run founder Mike Dove says that he has contacted shoe companies for product assistance but to no avail. My experience with shoe companies tells me there is still potential in this area.

Many shoe companies sponsor kids' running events. Some companies also donate shoes to needy children in Africa and other countries. Surely they can be tapped to help kids in America.

Kids' running shoes are a growing market, according to Lizzie Peterson, children's footwear buyer at Playmakers, a major retailer in Okemos, Michigan, that supports kids' events and programs such as the Michigan Mile and Feelin' Good Mileage Club. Peterson says that Asics, Adidas, Brooks, New Balance, and Nike are the major kids' brands. Sales have been so brisk that in September 2007 Playmakers opened a separate children's athletic footwear store adjacent to its main outlet.

Peterson's advice for parents purchasing children's shoes:

1. **Shoe choice.** Most kids choose shoes based on color and design. However, structural properties and comfort are critical. Parents should find a happy medium between a shoe's look and its support.

2. **Shoe use.** Kids should use running shoes only for running, not for other sports like tennis, soccer, or basketball, in which lateral movement requires different support. Using a tennis shoe for running can cause sprained ankles, says Dr. Kenneth Indahl, a Wall Township, New Jersey, podiatrist and triathlete.

3. **Shoe structure.** The better shoes have a wider top lip and more rubber around the toe for durability, as kids tend to scuff the front. They have a thin midsole, as kids are light and do not need the thick midsoles common in adult models. Shoes should not be so high off the ground, as greater height makes for instability. A number of companies use strong, duel-density foam for stability in the arch, to address fallen arches (that is, overpronation) and the fact that, inevitably, many kids will wear their running shoes for play.

4. **Shoe fit.** Kids' feet and legs do not grow at the same rate, says Dr. Brenda Armstrong, who instructs her Durham run-

ners (see chapter 5) to wear running shoes to avoid shin and ankle injuries. Lizzie Peterson says, "We always fit the larger foot so it's not crunched in. You can lace the smaller foot tighter. Some parents use an extra sock."

Both Peterson and Dr. Indahl say that cross-trainers are acceptable for children doing a few miles; these are heavier-duty shoes with properties similar to running shoes. They should not be used for long mileage or speed work.

To Dr. Indahl, what kids need most in a running shoe is biomechanical control—a good arch and firm heel counter to stabilize the feet, which are not structurally formed yet because of growth issues. He says that kids have a tendency toward tightness in the heel cords and calf muscles related to growth in the long bones in their legs, and inadequate footwear can exacerbate that problem.

Or young runners can go au naturel, as the speedy Kenyan children do, at least on occasion. "I'd like to see kids running barefoot on a nice, grassy area," says Dr. Bill Roberts. "Barefoot running builds up the muscles in the feet and lets feet do what they're supposed to do in developing."

▶ Is Your Child a "Star"?

No. Doctors specializing in youth sports and child development say that, despite what some parents may think, there is no such thing as an 8-, 9-, or 10-year-old "star" in running. Kids have all their development and maturity left. True talent and commitment are not genuine before puberty.

On the Run: A Primer for Ages 3 to 11

Starting out. Take your child to a running event with a kids' or family fun run, typically a mile or less. Parents can join in. Everyone can run or walk. Peer support is crucial. The perks, like wearing race numbers and getting postrun treats, will have any youngster asking for more.

Healthy fun. It's all about learning good health habits, making friends, and gently working young bodies. Kids' running should not dominate free time but fit in easily with a child's weekly schedule.

Must-do stretches. It's good to develop a running routine with a couple of exercises to be done before and after running. A couple of stretches will prime young bodies and serve to complete the activity afterward. Do 10 to 20 jumping jacks, which all kids love; have them count aloud. Also have them sit with legs extended and reach for their toes.

Fail-safe workouts. Go to a park or track where the child can do laps. Give the child a high five with each lap completed. If it's hot, spray them with a water bottle as they pass. Award stickers or other age-appropriate prizes for number of laps run.

Helpful parents. Network on the Web or through the community to find parent-supervised running groups or clubs for kids. They may be conducted by coaches, teachers, or just parents who run. You can always try to start a group yourself through the town, a school, a fitness center or YMCA, or perhaps a church or synagogue.

Running distances. Distances are expressed in yards, meters, or kilometers—for example, 100 yards (about the length of a city block), 400 meters (one lap of a track), 1,600 meters or a mile (four laps), and 5K (5 kilometers, which is 3.1 miles). The youngest kids do the shortest distances and can work up to a mile and more as they get older.

Age	Distance and Frequency
3–4	25 yards to 100 yards 1 to 2 days a week
5	50 yards to ¼ mile 1 to 2 days a week
6	100 yards to ½ mile 2 days a week
7	½ mile to 1 mile 2 days a week
8	½ mile to 2 miles 2 to 3 days a week
9	1 mile to 2 miles 2 to 3 days a week
10	1 mile to 3 miles 3 days a week
11	1 mile to 4–5 miles 3 days a week

Miles per week. One mile per week is a nice goal for young children. Older kids running two or three times a week can cover 5 to 10 miles. A preteen should not exceed 15 to 20 miles per week.

Racing by age. Many kids enjoy competing in races. Here are suggested race distances for children of various ages.

Age	Race Distance
3–4	25 to 100 yards
5	50 yards to ¼ mile
6	50 yards to ¼ mile
7	100 yards to 1 mile
8	100 yards to 1 mile
9	100 yards to 3K (1.8 miles)
10	100 yards to 5K (3.1 miles)
11	100 yards to 5K (3.1 miles)

Target mile times. While at this age running times should be deemphasized, they can help motivate youngsters and also satisfy those who become excited about running fast and improving their efforts. Here are some goal-oriented guidelines by age.

(continued)

Age	Target
7	11 to 12 minutes
8	10 to 11 minutes
9	9 to 10 minutes
10	8 to 9 minutes
11	7 to 8 minutes

3

Running with Young Racers

I see a turning point. Kids are enjoying running again. They feel so happy accomplishing something.

—Isabel Keeley, director of the Summer Nights
kids' running series in New Jersey

It's a sultry but exciting June evening at Battlefield State Park in Manalapan Township, New Jersey, with the first of six weekly events in the Freehold Area Running Club Summer Nights Running Series. The program, celebrating the twenty-fifth anniversary of its adult 5K (3.1-mile) run, boasts a popular series of youth races as well, and I'm anxious to see how this community effort is motivating kids to run and addressing childhood obesity. FARC, as we call it, is my local running club in central New Jersey, western Monmouth County, and I often hear neighborhood buzz about its kids' program, something of a pioneering effort when it began in 1993. At the time, the term "childhood obesity" was not making headlines, but the running community, usually ahead of the curve when it comes to health issues, felt that kids were in need of an extra push to get out and work their bodies. Club officer Isabel Keeley, a former FARC president, attended the Road Runners Clubs of America annual conventions in the early nineties and brought home some ideas from kids' running seminars. She took charge of the club's children's runs.

Isabel says that one idea she's carried through the years is to make sure the youngsters are given race numbers. While adults may take such numbers for granted, says Isabel, kids feel extra pride and enhanced self-esteem as part of a group. On this night, the number idea, even for the youngest kids, is a winner. Even toddlers beam with their new identity. And as I observe the large get-together on the park grounds, the numbers also serve to remind adults that the simplest things are often what grab kids the most.

Indeed, the act of parents pinning the race numbers to their youngsters' shirts seems to enthrall the children, perhaps as much as the running itself. I see kids mesmerized by parents' meticulous handling of safety pins and positioning of the rather large numbers on their small bodies; then, once the numbers are set, kids smile and check one another out, and some take off in a sprint as though to test their new prize. They have energy to burn and can't wait to use it.

For me, this scene is a revelation. I had not witnessed a FARC kids' race in years and before coming took note of the kids' sign-up flyer:

KIDS SUMMER NIGHTS RUNNING SERIES

June 20, 2007–August 8, 2007
Registration starts at 5:30 P.M.
Races start at 6:00 P.M.
At Battlefield State Park, Manalapan, N.J.
Sponsored by: Pauline's Health Food Stores
25 Yard Toddler Trot . . . 18 Months to 3 years
50 Yard Dash . . . 4 Years and Up

100 Yard Charge . . . 5 Years and Up
Half-Mile Race and Mile Race . . . 8 Years and Up
Ribbons and Ice Pops to All Finishers
T-Shirts and Trophies to Kids Who Pre-Enter for Series
Fee: $2.00 per Race or All Seven Races for $12.00

Earlier it was 95 degrees and humid. At 5:00 P.M., with the sun still blazing, I think there's no way that parents will take their kids out of air-conditioned comfort for an evening of vigorous exercise. And toddlers yet?

Race volunteers seem oblivious to the heat. They set up the finish line banner, timing apparatus, and PA system, the drinks and ice pops and T-shirts, the applications and race numbers, club banners, and other signage.

And the children come. Families pile out of the parking lot with kids of all ages in tow. Moms and dads push baby strollers. Youngsters clutch water bottles. Sisters and brothers hold hands. They scurry up to the registration tables to sign up. It looks like the first day of camp: low-key, informal, efficient, user-friendly.

The precious numbers are pinned on. Some are put on the child's chest (where they're supposed to go), others on the back. It really doesn't matter. As Isabel says, the numbers are used not for scoring but for pride. On the younger children, the numbers extend from chin to waist and even below. The kids wear T-shirts or tank tops. Some wear soccer or basketball jerseys. I notice some shirts that seem a little too heavy for the heat, in which thin fabrics and light colors are preferred.

Some parents are very fit-looking themselves and doing the adult 5K. In many cases, one or more parents is entered along with two or three children in a full-blown family fitness outing, a growing trend at big-city marathons and apparently in Monmouth County, New Jersey, as well. Parents lug coolers with drinks and goodies. Here and there are overweight parents who would do well to follow their children's examples. But fit or not, all parents appear to act in the spirit of the event, which stresses participation and healthy fun over time and place.

BUILDING GOOD HABITS

The main goal is building good habits for the long term. I ask a local high school coach, Bob Andrews, who's using the adult 5K event as an easy workout for his cross-country team, about the kids' races. He's entered his own son, Robby, over the years, and now as a teenager Robby is a high school all-American. "This is an opportunity to experience the sport and get comfortable with it," he says. "Everybody's a winner here. There's no discouragement, only encouragement. The prize is the ice pop."

With that incentive, the field will only grow. Isabel tells me that 250 kids are signed up for the entire series, and she expects another 50 or more the next week. The word is spread through the club Web site and also via flyers distributed at the district schools. With a bullhorn, she encourages parents to make sure their kids drink and stay cool and pace themselves during the runs. "It's about finishing," she says.

In the hubbub of kids darting in all directions, I'm not sure how much attention is being paid to the heat issue. What safeguards must we take with children? When I check with Dr. Brenda Armstrong, associate professor of pediatrics and pediatric cardiology at Duke University School of Medicine, who is also a coach and team doctor with a youth track squad, she tells me that in fact kids can handle heat as long as precautions are taken. She says that kids should have minimum exposure to sunlight before and after competing, wear lightweight, loose-fitting clothes, and drink a minimum of eight glasses of water on hot days.

Running Children and the Heat

Children running and racing in the heat should take the following precautions, according to Dr. Brenda Armstrong, associate professor of pediatrics and pediatric cardiology at Duke University School of Medicine and a coach of the Durham Striders youth track team, which often trains and competes in hot conditions.

1. At track meets or running events lasting several hours, they should stay in the shade when not competing and avoid direct sunlight from 10 A.M. to 4 P.M.
2. They should drink fluids hourly even if they're not thirsty. They should drink enough to want to go to the bathroom at least once every three to four hours.
3. Fluid intake should total at least 64 ounces of water in a twenty-four-hour period.
4. They should drink water while warming up for an event, and immediately after the event.
5. They should wear loose-fitting clothes and light colors.

There are three types of heat illness:

- **Heat cramps** are short-lived but severe cramps in the leg and arm muscles and abdomen, and occur because of inadequate fluid intake in the context of vigorous exercise. They require no more than a cool place to rest and fluids.
- **Heat exhaustion** is more serious and tends to occur after prolonged exposure to heat and lack of fluids. Symptoms include dehydration (dry tongue, no sweating, no need to urinate), fatigue, weakness, headache, nausea, vomiting. Immediately put the child in a cooler environment and

give her fluids; remove her clothing and put her in a tepid/cool (but not cold) bath and watch her carefully. If she is disoriented in any way and cannot take in fluids, she should be taken to a hospital emergency room immediately for IV fluid hydration and care.

- **Heat stroke** is the most serious and life-threatening. It occurs when heat illness is inadequately treated and body temperature rises quickly (to as high as 106 degrees), which can lead to brain damage, seizures, and death. Prolonged exercise in the heat with inadequate fluid intake can lead to heat stroke. Immediate medical care is necessary.

Before the races start, most families congregate in the small area of shade where club officials answer questions. As race time nears, kids limber up, coached by older siblings or parents. Stretching exercises seem to be hit or miss. Young children running short distances in a fun-run atmosphere do not need a lot of stretching. But a little loosening up makes sense, and why not introduce good habits for later on? The gathering presents a wonderful opportunity for FARC to organize a child-centered group stretching regimen that could be another highlight of the evening. The routine could be listed on the schedule—say, at 5:45, "stretching for all ages"—and led by a high school athlete or adult runner with an instinct for tickling kids' funny bones. Choose three or four easy-to-follow exercises and make a game out of it, like Simon Says. Or do a spelling bee during the routine, asking who can spell "hamstring" and "muscle" and "stretching." Maybe the leader can wear a funny hat. Give out flyers with the diagrams of the stretches so the youngsters can practice at home (and improve their spelling), or put them on the club Web site. Use the time, when presumably you'd have the kids' attention, to reinforce important running concepts: don't start out too fast, pace yourself, run in a straight line, don't look back; it's okay to stop and walk if you have to.

But many parents rush over from work and there are some crowd management issues with the large turnout. "We've really increased our numbers," Isabel tells me. "Almost double since last year." She adds, "I see a turning point. Kids are enjoying running again. They feel so happy accomplishing something."

And there's no better place to do it than at Battlefield, a historic site with broad meadows where the Battle of Monmouth was staged on June 28, 1778. It was the longest battle of the Revolutionary War and resulted in a major victory for General George Washington and the Continental Army. The site, 1,818 acres, remains pristine and, I must say, fairly underutilized given the growth of our area. Whenever I come here to run, I see no more than a handful of people walking their dogs.

KIDS RARING TO GO

But tonight it's showtime with upward of 250 kids ready to run, race numbers ready, and hundreds of parents supporting them. From the meadow where the youngest kids race, you can look out to the broad plain, lush fields of corn, and apple orchards that meet the clear blue sky, a brilliant setting on this hazy summer night when barely a leaf moves.

Lindsey Golotko, a 7-year-old second grader in Freehold Township, can't wait to get started. She's doing the half mile; she says she practices running in her cul-de-sac and learned how to pump her arms from her older sister. Lindsey wears number 947. Her mother, Jodi, tells me, "She likes the T-shirt, likes doing something her sister does. She's hoping to get a trophy." I refer to her older daughter's running, prompting Mom to say, "They just look great when they run."

It's natural for young children to follow their older siblings into running, and that's evident throughout the park. The leader of the pack is Tom Apostle of Freehold Borough, who has all six of his youngsters running. The oldest, Roy, is a 15-year-old sophomore on the Freehold cross-country team. Roy was among the event's early participants in the mid-nineties. "I don't think we've missed a summer," says Tom.

The sibling pattern is also pivotal in the upper echelons of teenage running. Many of the better high school track and cross-country teams around the nation have two or more siblings running at the same time and a steady flow of several children following one another over a period of years. In New Mexico, for example, state and national power Los Alamos High has seen five Sandoval children of parents Anthony and Mary come through its program. A number of the Sandoval brood went on to excel on college teams. In fall 2007, Pennsylvania state girls' champion Emmaus High was bolstered by sophomore triplets Amanda, Christina, and Brianna Faust.

This is important for parents to know: get one child out running and others will likely follow, and soon the entire family will be involved in a healthy endeavor with many benefits beyond the running. The feel-good effects of running facilitate better family relationships, according to psychologists, who note that young runners tend to be more confident and less vulnerable to peer pressure than their nonrunning classmates.

The discipline that running teaches, along with the many good habits, helps kids figure out "who they are and where they fit in," according to Joel Fish, Ph.D., director of the Center for Sports Psychology in Philadelphia. Running can be particularly beneficial, says Fish, for the insecure child who lacks confidence.

Bob Andrews, the high school coach, feels the same. In addition to his son, Robby, he's had a daughter running and she is now on a college team. He feels that running has grounded his kids, who have followed a mature, wholesome path undeterred by teen pressures and the style of the moment.

LEARNING TO LOOK STRAIGHT AHEAD

All of tonight's kids have the same opportunity. I approach another parent, Charmaine Chestnut, whose 7-year-old son, Garrett, is doing the 25-, 50-, and 100-yard events. I address Garrett.

How often do you run?
Garrett: **Many times.**
What have you learned about running?
Garrett: **Don't look left, right, or behind.**
What's the best thing about running?
Garrett: **When you get to the end.**

Garrett also plays peewee football and is running with knee pads because he has football practice later on. "This is our second year in the kids' running program," says mom. "Garrett's fast and loves racing older kids. I tell him he'll get better and faster if he sticks with it."

Another benefit of the five-race menu is that kids can easily do more than one event. The age guideline is just that: a guideline, not a hard rule. The informal mix allows for different ages to join in, and with so much spirit in the air there's no risk of a slower child feeling out of touch. Kids seem to like many options and try different events from week to week. The five races also reduce each field to a manageable size, ensuring that kids won't fall in a crush of bodies and hurt themselves, and the many events spread out the talent, so the chance of a ringer winning everything is unlikely. In addition, boys and girls have their own single-sex races in the younger age groups.

The 25-yard Toddler Trot is called. Isabel announces, "Mommies and daddies can run with your children. Older brothers and sisters can run with little brothers and sisters." Some parents and siblings take the offer. Isabel commands the bullhorn and with a teacherlike approach shows the kids how to line up and make sure their shoelaces are tied. She asks for all eyes to be on her and tells the group to wait for instructions before running. "When you line kids up," Isabel tells me, "you're working on their attention span."

It's doubtful a group of toddlers ever stood in one place for so long. For some, it's just impossible. One girl leans forward with hands on knees and darts ahead. Isabel gently grabs her by the shoulders and ushers her back.

Finally it's time, and Isabel makes it official: "Ready, set, go!" About fifteen girls dash across the field. Some run, some walk; some laugh, one or two cry. Two girls run holding hands. One has her number on the front, the other on the back. The oldest club volunteers, men in their 70s, hold the finish tape, actually string.

"Running teaches a lot," Isabel says. "More than fitness."

Then the boys line up. They're edgy, jumping ahead. Isabel is firm. "Never look at the starter," she calls out. "Look straight ahead toward the finish. Listen to my voice." Girls from the first race join in to run again. "Go." They tear ahead in a jumble of bodies. One boy reaches the finish, turns around, and runs back to the start. A girl decides to run backward from the finish to the start, then run normally to the finish. It may be organized, but in a toddler world, it's also deliciously spontaneous.

The 50-yard takes the stage. Girls first, then boys. "Make a straight line," Isabel says. That seems too much to ask of these mostly prekindergarten kids. Isabel delivers her starter's "ready, set, go" routine, and as the field zigzags to the waiting senior citizen finish crew, I ask Isabel if kids really need a formal start like that. She says she does it so they'll know what to expect when they compete as older runners. I'm still not convinced, but I do know that children like routines, and familiar instructions can serve as behavioral cues each time they take part.

There must be a hundred kids total running the 50-yarders. Some fly right through the finish, while others run tentatively, looking at their feet. I go up to the first-place girl, Juliana, an 8-year-old third grader from Freehold who plays soccer.

What's the best part about running?
Juliana: Running.

GET YOUR ICE POPS!

"Everyone," bellows Isabel, "there's ice pops! Get your ice pops!" The youngsters slurp all flavors—lime, orange, raspberry—ice pop in one hand, finish ribbon in the other hand. It's a big night for Kathy Springer-Heller and her husband, Joel. Their kids, Drew, 3, and Kathy, almost 5, are getting ready for the 100 yards after doing the 25 and 50. I talk with the parents.

Dad: During the day, they ask, "Is tonight the races?"
Mom: They love the ribbons.
Dad: They don't just come for the Popsicle. They know what it's about. It's an event for them.
Mom: It's not video games.
Dad: It's getting out and running and keeping active. Enjoying the outdoors.

Drew wears funny, oversized sunglasses and number 990. Kathy, holding a teddy bear, wears number 989.

The 100 is run on a steep hill. The youngsters' age range looks like 3 to 9, from half-pints to growing preteens. Isabel addresses the girls' lineup as "ladies." I think that some basic instruction on how to run uphill—lean forward from the hips; shorten your stride; pump arms up and back, not side to side—would benefit the older kids. Isabel repeats that parents can run along with their little ones. The "charge" lives up to its name. Despite the challenging incline, most of the kids are able to race with no letup to the finish. I see some of the stragglers laughing their way up. Most of the kids don't "break" the finish string but duck under it.

The half mile takes place in the parking lot. About fifty kids and a dozen parents line up. "Does everyone know the course?" shouts club president John Weitz, who will lead the field by bike. One father gives his son a good-luck kiss on the forehead; another pours water on his son's head and neck, a great idea. I think that someone should be spraying all the kids at the start.

"Quiet at the start," insists Isabel. She checks race numbers. Very few youngsters wear hats for sun protection. Perhaps there should be club guidelines insisting on that, like helmets in a bike race. "If you start to get hot, walk," instructs Isabel. "If you get a stitch in your side, put your hands over your head, let oxygen get into your lungs, take a deep breath, and walk till the stitch goes away." Too complicated? Maybe just tell them to walk and breathe deeply. More instruction from Isabel: "When you finish you're going to get a place card; go to the desk and hand it in."

Just then a father does a Clark Kent change of work clothes into running togs to join his daughter.

FAST STARTERS NEED PATIENCE

Despite all the pacing admonitions, a bunch of boys flies out in sprinting mode. This is comparable to first-time soccer players swarming around the ball no matter what coaches say about spreading out. Can anything be done about the impatient racers? Perhaps by telling the entire field to walk for thirty seconds, then ease into the race. It's worth a try.

One 8-year-old girl who places fourth profits from this approach. "I jogged the first half, then ran the second half," she tells me. Her mother says her daughter had expressed a fear of competition. "She was worried about running a race. She has a thing about winning. If she's not first, it's a problem, because she's good in other sports," the mother explains. "I told her, 'Go out and have fun, you're a good athlete, you got plenty of sleep last night . . . just do your best.'"

Joel Fish, the psychologist, believes that parents can take pressure off children at races by getting them to express feelings. He says there are three emotional skills involved for the child: knowing the feeling, assessing it, and expressing it.

Some kids may not wear their emotions on the sleeves, but food coloring, yes. I see the half-mile winner devouring a tricolor ice pop. He's Brandon Mazzarella of Manalapan, age 12, chalking up his first victory. "It felt good," he says. "At the end I got a little tired. I could have paced myself better." Considering the boy's maturity, I ask Brandon if he feels motivated to run more. "Not right now," he says. "Maybe tomorrow."

Brandon's 11-year-old brother, Joseph, was third. Previously, he ran the sprints. This is his first half mile. "In the summer I get fat," he says. "I'm trying to keep my weight down."

Since the Mazzarella boys seem eager to talk, I probe further, asking Joseph what he thinks about on the starting line. "That I hope she [Isabel] speaks loudly because one time I couldn't hear her and I got a late start." What do other youngsters need to know about running? "Stretch, have fun; after the race when you get an ice pop, eat slowly so you can enjoy it."

The boys say they got interested in running from doing soccer and gymnastics and seeing their mother run on a treadmill.

You can't beat parental example. Bert Lundberg comes for the 5K and brings 6-year-old Nicholas for the half mile. "I'm not really training him. I don't even know his times. He says he likes it. I don't force it," says the father. Laura Donovan also comes for the 5K with a daughter in the mile and warns, "Don't push them too much. You don't want to strain their bodies while they're developing, and you don't want them to burn out mentally either."

The issue of young kids overdoing it is never far away. A FARC member comes over to me and says, "You see that girl, 9? I'm training a 9-year-old." I say, "You're *training* a 9-year-old?" He replies, "The father asked me to, and it's a good thing, because the father was overdoing it. He had his daughter doing 3-to-4-mile runs every day. I cut her back to a mile and a half three times a week."

CHEERING WITHOUT SCREAMING

Overzealous track parents grate on Isabel, who tells me, "They are trying to live through their kids. The kids run harder before it's time. Some parents scream at their kids to run faster. They should go run a mile themselves and see how their legs ache and breathing is labored and maybe then they won't be so quick to yell at their kids."

The screaming parent, at least this night, is the exception rather than the rule. But it's also the case that many parents, especially nonrunners, don't know quite how to handle their running kids. Their context usually is soccer or basketball, where screaming is the norm.

Some forty youngsters and about fifteen parents line up for the mile, the longest and climactic kids' event, two loops of the half-mile course. I mill around asking parents for brief comments, and most tell me they're "new to this." As a response, FARC may need to be more proactive in educating parents. That may lessen the chances of parents overtraining their 9-year-olds or screaming at them to run faster.

Isabel herself offers a dose of smart postrace parenting. "After the race," she says, "tell them they did a good job and ask them how they felt. Don't give your opinion so fast. Get their feedback, which may be different from what parents think or assume." If they're old enough, she adds, give them responsibility for their running, like choosing the next week's event.

With the sun still searing, the mile winner, a boy, comes running across the finish in 6 minutes 35 seconds. The first girl, Ciara Roche, runs 7 minutes even. She's 9. Her father was once a noted runner. I speak with her mom, Nancy, also a runner. "She did well in the school Presidential Fitness Challenge," mom tells me. "We try and teach her to be a good athlete, to pace herself and learn from her experience."

When I question Ciara, she is articulate beyond her years. She explains her racing strategy and how she learns about different courses and where to accelerate and make moves. I realize that a race not only enables kids to learn about running but also requires critical thinking, some math and geography, and even a bit of science. Distance, hills, weather, how the body works: it's an all-in-one experience, the best kind of learning for real life. Not only that, but you have fun doing it, and the only homework is more running.

Even with all that constructive joy, the best part for any child, as 9-year-old Ciara affirms, is "when you finish."

▶ Race Numbers, Ice Pops, and Good Listening

1. First races. Youngsters can start running as young as toddlers in kiddie dashes as a prelude to longer races as they get older. Early involvement builds good habits and makes running seem natural. Kids see other children doing the same.

2. Repeat performance. The best programs are those with a number of events throughout the year so children have continuity and try to improve and feel better with each succeeding race.

3. A running habit. Young kids starting out don't need formal training but should run a little here and there to stay in shape, especially for a longer event like a quarter mile or half mile, while also doing other sports or activities.

4. Family fitness. When parents and siblings participate, it builds long-term reinforcement while making the endeavor a family fitness feast.

5. Creature comforts. Kids thrive on accoutrements like wearing race numbers, earning prizes, and having rewarding snacks afterward (include fruit in your goody bag, as opposed to candy or donuts).

6. Beating the heat. On hot days, doctors advise drinking several glasses of water in the course of the day and finding shade at the race site before and after running. Also, wear light, comfortable clothing.

7. Learning experience. Use the races to encourage learning about the body, listening to instructions, an understanding of distance and time, feeling comfortable in large groups, and proper pacing.

8. Priority on fun. Encourage fun and participation, not performance; with consistency and growth, improvements will come.

9. Lookin' good. Cheer proudly for your youngsters, but try not to scream for them to "run faster."

10. Role models. Give older youngsters some responsibility, like showing a younger sibling what to do, being in charge of the water bottles, and helping to decide which events to run next.

4

Running with Healthy Schools

On spring break, I want you to run. If you run only from the fridge to the couch, that's not enough.

—RICH DEXTER, VIRGINIA PE TEACHER WHOSE
STUDENTS EXCEL IN AN ANNUAL FUN RUN

What makes for a healthy school? What are the important factors that inspire schoolchildren to enjoy running, show vigor, and develop ideas about fitness and well-being that will benefit all aspects of their young lives?

What has enabled one school in Springfield, Virginia—Lynbrook Elementary—to win the Healthy School award at the Marine Corps Marathon in the Washington, D.C., area all seven years since the accolade began to recognize participation in the event's Healthy Kids Fun Run?

It can't be a fancy school building or elaborate facilities, because when I visit the school one early spring day I find a rather drab, boxy exterior and modest playground. It can't be an affluent school population with families that patronize health clubs, because Lynbrook is a Title 1 school in which more than 60 percent of the students are entitled to free lunch. It can't be the kids' spiffy running gear, because most children run in heavy basketball sneakers or even street shoes. It can't be the cultural impetus of status-driven children's achievement, because there are more than forty nationalities among the 400 students, many parents are enrolled in ESL classes, and while the Beltway is nearby, this community is as far outside it as you can get.

And surely it can't be the luxury of daily physical education classes, because like most schools, Lynbrook meets only a minimum requirement, as prescribed by Fairfax County and handed down by the state, of at least 60 minutes of PE a week. The principal, Mary McNamee, provides two 30-minute periods for students in kindergarten through sixth grade. She says that PE falls under a time umbrella linked with music and art and that, in addition, issues of space and staffing intervene. After all, she has only 1.4 PE teachers in the building.

So how could it be that, despite these handicaps, in October 2007 Lynbrook had its biggest turnout yet—172 entrants, more than half the eligible students—in the Healthy Kids Fun Run, a 1-mile race staged in the Pentagon parking lot? Parents paid the $2 entry fee, and all 172 kids, boys and girls age 8 to 12 in grades two through six, showed up on time wearing Lynbrook Leprechauns T-shirts, filled three buses, got their official race numbers, were accompanied by seventeen teacher-chaperones, and completed the mile run as parents cheered and wept and the Marines ran from behind to make sure no child went astray.

"We don't leave anyone on the battlefield, and we don't leave any kid on the race course," says Rick Nealis, a retired career officer and race director of both the Marines' fun run and the megamarathon held the next day.

HEALTHY STUDENTS LEARN TO RUN

As Lynbrook is a model for schools—even those with little re-sources—seeking to improve kids' health with running as a linch-pin, the Healthy Kids Fun Run is definitive in charting the explosive growth in youth running, especially with its tie-in to a major urban marathon. The Marine Corps Marathon began in 1976 with 1,175 runners and is now capped at about 21,000. When the online entry period is announced every spring, the event typically fills up in ten days.

Nealis got the idea for a kids' run in 2000 when he was stunned by the poor showing of American marathoners at the Sydney Olympics. The only U.S. man to meet the Olympic quali-fying time that year finished sixty-ninth. Likewise, only one U.S. woman qualified for the Games, placing nineteenth.

Among runners, the marathon is seen as a symbol of national endurance, a touchstone of a people's get-up-and-go, and Nealis, prodded in part by his military background, felt that young Amer-icans were going soft. He wrote up a position paper for his Ma-rine superiors on the weakening state of youth fitness while advocating a children's fun run. "To instill all the values we put into the marathon," says Nealis. "Get kids into the sport. Ener-gize them. The generals bought into it. The first year, 2000, we had about 300 kids with very little promotion."

By 2004 the fun run field had grown to over 1,300 and Nealis had to create three divisions, or "waves," by age bracket (6–7, 8–9, 10–13) for safety reasons and course management. By 2007 the field had swelled to almost 2,000, and Nealis expected 3,000 for fall 2008. Standing last October with the top brass in a sea of sweating children at the finish, one elder colonel gasped to Nea-lis in awe of what their event had become.

As the students gather at Lynbrook, I begin to get an inkling of what moves the young Leprechauns. Indeed, it is Leprechaun Day at the school, the Friday before spring break, with St. Patrick's Day three days away. Few students are Irish, but the occasion is a tradition held annually since the school opened in 1957. Even with the holiday spirit featuring green outfits and games, students parade through the building in orderly fashion, lugging heavy book bags and with a certain educational intent on their faces.

It's also a noteworthy day in the gym, as PE teacher Richard Dexter is conducting his monthly running challenge, the Fitnessgram Pacer Test. The gym is festooned with ornate, homemade Healthy Kids Fun Run award banners and the flags of at least forty nations representing the diversity of the student body. A U.S. map is affixed to the far wall. Dexter sports a curly green wig in honor of the day, drawing approving smiles from Kimberly Clancy, the physical education supervisor of Fairfax County's 137 elementary schools, who has come for a brief observational visit.

A fourth-grade class plus some sixth graders who missed the test the other day march into the well-lighted gymnasium. The kids, thirty strong, sit on their designated spots. Dexter reviews the procedures with a booming voice, high expectations, and a sense of humor.

"All set?"

"Yes!" the youngsters respond.

"Do *not* let me down," he implores.

HEALTHY STUDENTS USE MIND AND BODY

The kids dash to the wall with the map for warm-ups. While doing jumping jacks they recite states and capitals—boys call out states and girls respond with capitals, then they switch. Each rhythmic movement has a geography tag. Then they use the wall while stretching calves, hamstrings, and quadriceps muscles. When Dexter refers aloud to the "gastroc," the children know that he means the gastrocnemious, a muscle in the calf. Then it's back to the floor for seated arm raises and more stretches such as toe touches as the children call out the vowels, "A . . . E . . . I . . . O . . . U . . . and sometimes Y," and Dexter booms, "Butt, groin, hams . . ."

Integrating regular subject matter into fitness—what Dexter calls "cross-curriculum"—shows children that learning is one continuum and that calisthenics, running, geography, and language all work together in developing mind, body, and pride. These kids eat it up.

This same integrative approach has generated running excitement at Carmel River Elementary School in California, which, like Lynbrook, has a student body of 400 and, also like Lynbrook, has had the largest number of schoolchildren (more than 100 at last count) in a favorite local event, the Big Sur 5K. The principal, Jay Marden, says that his teachers find ways to merge math, history, science, geography, and language arts with running. The laps and miles run are used in math lessons. Distance covered is used in map skills and geography. The students write essays about their running experiences.

"If we get kids running around a half mile a day, that's a good starting point," says Marden, recently named Principal of the Year in California. "Some need a kick in the pants to get going."

Or a booming, passionate voice. There are two groups in the Lynbrook gym, those doing the Pacer Test and those on the sidelines keeping a lap tally. Dexter's command fills the gym as it will all day: "Prepare yourself to get a new personal best."

The children's precision would impress the Marines. But after all, Dexter, 38, grew up an army brat—his father, a West Point graduate, was a career military man who did two tours in Vietnam and served at the Pentagon. Dexter played football at the University of Richmond and before getting started in teaching spent eighteen months in Antarctica providing logistical support for the National Science Foundation, braving −100° wind chills.

His students will not starve for discipline. But they seem to like discipline and responsibility. They eagerly pair off with partners, each runner with a scorekeeper. Dexter distributes recording sheets and pencils. A sign states: "Get FIT: Frequency, Intensity, Training."

"Runners, stand up!" The kids take their positions on one side of the gym, on the basketball endline, preparing to run the prescribed 20-meter laps (about 66 feet) to the other baseline. I express surprise that kids as young as 9 can be counted on to accurately record the data. No problem, says Rich. Those kids won't let him down either.

HEALTHY STUDENTS ACHIEVE PERSONAL BESTS

Dexter has all the students' test records in a computer program linked to a PowerPoint presentation that appears on a big screen. A program voice begins, "The Fitnessgram Pacer Test is a multistage aerobics capacity test that progressively gets more difficult as it continues. The 20-meter Pacer Test will begin in thirty seconds. Line up at the start. The running speeds start slowly but get faster. Every time you hear the signal, a single lap should be completed. Remember to run in a straight line and for as long as possible. The second time you fail to complete a lap before the sound, the test is over."

Dexter is high on the test because it is ideally suited to everything he teaches kids about pacing themselves, making month-to-month progress, and taking ownership of their health. The youngsters do not compete against other children and are not held to any conceptualized standard; the test, used nationwide, has minimum levels based on laps run that Dexter refers to but does not dwell on. The kids' only mission, as Dexter frames it, is to try hard and, as often as they can, improve by just one lap to achieve a personal best. The kids can't "lose" unless they goof off or ignore instructions. "Pace, not race," Dexter repeats.

You cannot become much of a runner if you start out too fast, develop shortness of breath or muscle pain, and have to stop. But kids are impulsive, get excited, and follow others. It takes discipline, confidence, and understanding to follow Dexter's orders. This is the seventh month of school, the seventh Pacer Test, and by now most kids get it.

Dexter shows me the chart with every student's personal best. The kids all know their scores. Every child in third through sixth grades also has a fitness portfolio with lap tallies for each year, other exercise data, and goals. Dexter pulls out the record of a sixth-grade girl whom he regards as a disappointment. "She did 26 laps in third grade. She's still doing 26 laps," he says. "She does the minimum." Dexter says that preteen girls can be a tough sell. Some are already developing, wear makeup, and flirt.

Music plays, the first beep sounds, and the kids start running. Most trot along at proper pace, up and back across the gym to the rhythm of the beeps. Few kids rest for a moment after each lap as they're supposed to; this tires them faster. No one wears real running shoes; they all have generic sneakers. "If they're not wearing leather," says Rich, "I'm happy." He tells me that one second-grade girl "ran like a gazelle" in patent leather shoes.

Half the group is still running after 30 laps. Three boys remain at 40. One of them runs in a jacket. Two remain at 45. One, a soccer player named Oscar, stops at 50 and darts to the floor to lie down. The last man standing, Kendall, a 10-year-old fourth grader wearing a Denver Nuggets jersey, does 61 laps (about three-quarters of a mile) before stopping. A personal best!

"I feel great because I waited all year to achieve this goal," Kendall tells me. He's been doing the Pacer Test since kindergarten, plays baseball, and basketball, and feels "running goes with it."

HEALTHY STUDENTS ARE TAUGHT
UNITY AND TOLERANCE

Another day I speak with Kendall's dad, also named Kendall and a runner too. He says his son is stress-free from running and "doesn't let things bother him." The father lauds Lynbrook's efforts, pointing out how well youngsters from many different backgrounds get along. "Running helps with that," he says.

After Kendall's personal best, Rich Dexter exclaims, "I'm fired up!" That's the phrase he uses every time a child excites him by working hard. He adds, "There's only so much I can do two days a week. I'm hoping they can draw on this memory and translate it into the real world. I hope I'm building life skills as well as love of running."

Dexter is the 0.4 part of the Lynbrook PE staff. He teaches two days a week while caring for his three children the other days. His wife works full-time in human resources. The full-time Lynbrook PE teacher is Jed Bobier, who this day is wrapped up in Leprechaun Day. Instead of filling out Dexter's position with an additional teacher, Lynbrook, as principal McNamee says, allots as much time as it can.

Relentless academic testing, amid No Child Left Behind dictates, dominates the educational landscape. While childhood obesity is at least as much a national calamity as deficiencies in reading or math are, it's almost fruitless politics to lobby for more PE. In the vicious cycle of distorted priorities, severe cuts in PE (and even recess time) have contributed to the proliferation of overweight children.

Kimberly Clancy, the Fairfax County PE supervisor, who serves on a state coalition to fight childhood obesity, says most of her schools do the same 60 minutes a week of PE as Lynbrook does. A few do 80 or 90 minutes. For more, she says, parents must play a role outside of school. That takes time, energy, and knowledge. At Lynbrook, McNamee says, "Our families work two and three jobs to finance their rent and necessities of life." The school does what it can for parents, like coordinating fitness nights and, through community agencies, providing scholarships for a handful of students to attend camp.

With limited PE, educators often seek supplemental programs. In New Jersey, Patricia Gasparini, the principal of Woodruff Elementary in Berkeley Heights and a runner, started a Happy Feet Club in which close to 100 children in second through fifth grades—nearly half the student body—meet one afternoon a week for running. They have individual and group goals, and many kids participate in a 5K race. Also in New Jersey, at St. Mary's School in Middletown, a PE teacher and a track coach got more than 150 children in a student body of 675 to join a Marathon Kids program for twice-a-week running. Nearby, Brielle Elementary School started a student mileage club with rewards for every quarter mile walked or run during lunch period.

With equal zeal, a Kalispell, Montana, PE teacher, Ross Darner, obtained a federal Physical Education Program (PEP) grant for $90,000 to create a fitness room and summer program that in its first year had almost one-half of the area's fifth and sixth graders running and doing other workouts. Darner found blood pressure reduced in those kids completing the program.

HEALTHY STUDENTS NEED COMMUNITY SUPPORT

The success of some grassroots school running programs has led to corporate sponsorship and greater numbers still. In Flint, Michigan—Michael Moore's infamously poor hometown—the CrimFit Youth Programs, an array of running events involving 8,000 students in every one of the city's public elementary schools, has a roster of sponsors including Sam's Club and the Ruth Mott Foundation. The youth program began as a modest offshoot of a popular adult road race, the Bobby Crim 10-Miler. The Go! St. Louis Read, Right, and Run Marathon, part of a multifaceted Family Fitness Weekend with many children's programs, has nineteen sponsors led by Saturn and Whole Foods.

Serving a different population, the Marathon Project in Dutchess County, north of New York City, pairs adult running mentors with at-risk youth in the Poughkeepsie and Beacon school districts. The after-school program for kids as young as 7 is organized by the Mid-Hudson Road Runners Club and trains the older teenage participants for races as long as a half-marathon.

Surveys show that a disproportionate number of Latino and African American children are overweight and obese. That makes Lynbrook's running program all the more essential. As McNamee says, "We have to provide a healthy, nurturing environment. They can't be learners if we don't provide that." How can she tell if the running really works? "There's qualitative and quantitative data," she says. "We get qualitative. When the children come back from PE, they are energized, their self-esteem is high and they are available for learning."

Dexter's bear-hug embrace extends beyond the monthly Pacer Tests to half-mile and mile runs he conducts four times a year as well as a climactic Dream Mile featuring the fastest kids at the end of the term and a full-school turnout to cheer. He preaches continuity, no down time, no stopping. He doesn't mind kids pushing so hard for a personal best that, in a rare case, a child loses his lunch in the gym. He hates the summer, when kids leave his grasp and fitness levels tend to drop off.

HEALTHY STUDENTS RESPOND TO A PE DREAM TEAM

Dexter says he's not reinventing the wheel but learning from others. Lynbrook's Healthy Kids Fun Run tradition began in 2001 with another PE teacher, Christy Yang, a marathoner who'd also used the Pacer Test and took about a dozen student-runners to the D.C. event as a field trip. She had no idea there was an award for school participation.

The next year Yang was joined at Lynbrook by Sean Niehoff, with Dexter coming in part-time a year after that. The trio worked together as a PE dream team. Yang then left to care for her first child. Niehoff, a full-timer, worked with Dexter through June 2006, when he left for Eagle View, a new school in the district.

Niehoff set up the same PE and running program there, also entering Eagle View in the Healthy Kids Fun Run. Last fall, the school set a record with 195 runners; with an enrollment of 700, Eagle View was declared the large-schools winner, with Lynbrook's title coming in the medium-size category. Barrett Elementary of Alexandria, Virginia, was the small-schools winner with 114 runners, giving Fairfax County a sweep. Dexter and Niehoff both say they nurture a friendly rivalry "for the health of the kids."

Niehoff, 33, has built-in motivation. He's a wheelchair athlete who the last two years, after spending an exhausting day with the kids on a Saturday, rolled the Marine Corps Marathon on Sunday. In 2007, he improved his time by 45 minutes to 3:27. Niehoff brings his racing chairs to school to show the students. That's part of his "linking" process, giving youngsters a broader context for their efforts.

A smart PE teacher knows how to tap students' abundant energy. Dexter ends every class with tag games in which kids run around the gym practically nonstop to 1950s rock tunes. Then the children sit on their spots in a blissful stupor listening to Dexter's stump speech: "On spring break, I hope you will run or do something other than video games. If you run only from the fridge to the couch, that's not enough, ladies and gentlemen."

Then a sixth-grade class enters the gym, sits, and, to Dexter's prodding, repeats: "We can do it! We can do it!" Warm-ups, states

and capitals, arms and vowels, runners and partners. These older
kids talk and laugh as they start their laps. Their chart shows a
previous lap range from 16 to 77. "Go . . . go . . . go . . ." The first
casualty comes at 24 laps. Dexter points out the sixth-grade girl
who's disappointed him. "C'mon, girl!" She stops at 27, a personal best by one lap. Eureka! There are four kids alive at 50
laps. The last one gives in at 63.

Mayra, wearing jeans, nails a personal best with 52. How
about those jeans? "Comfortable," she says. Yorshua, wearing a
"Kiss Me, I'm Irish" button," nails a personal best with 35. He
tells me he's lost four pounds.

Then tag, oldies, running, droopy contentment. And the
speech: "Whoever ran the Healthy Kids Fun Run, stand up."
More than half rise. (And the numbers continue to rise as Lynbrook's turnout in 2008 is 255 students, a 50 percent increase.)
"This is the first day of the rest of your life. Get off your butt and
get moving if you want a personal best next month."

HEALTHY STUDENTS THRIVE ON FITNESS GOALS

The Pacer Test, one of a battery of tests in the Fitnessgram menu
(there are thirteen tests for aerobic capacity, body composition,
muscular strength, endurance, and flexibility for teachers to
choose from) is not actually a fitness program but an assessment.
Approved for Virginia schools by the state's Department of Education, Fitnessgram was created in 1982 by the Cooper Institute
for Aerobics Research.

Initially, Fitnessgram used a single test already in existence.
Within five years, the institute came up with its first round of signature tests. In 1992, the Pacer Test, developed by Canadian exercise physiologists at the University of Montreal, was added to
the Fitnessgram program. It is one of three aerobic capacity tests.
The others are a mile run and mile walk. Eventually software

was added. The materials, still owned by Cooper, are published and sold by Human Kinetics. A software package with data entry for students that produces a complete report sells for $319 per school. The Pacer Test alone with a CD and manual sells for $29.

Fitnessgram is currently used by at least 20,000 schools and school districts nationwide, according to Marilu D. Meredith, national project director since the program's inception. Some states, such as Texas and California, mandate it. Some large school districts, including those in Houston and Los Angeles, also require it. Meredith said there's no way to know which of the thirteen tests are used in particular schools.

Meredith also said that upward of 700 schools in New York City are using Fitnessgram and "making tremendous strides" in PE. At least some of those strides result from a multitiered New York Road Runners Foundation program in which 30,000 students in 100-plus elementary schools run in Mighty Milers clubs, over 2,000 youngsters in more than 60 middle schools participate on Young Runners teams, and schoolkids of all ages are engaged in City Sports track programs throughout the year.

The Canadian researchers determined the effectiveness of the Pacer Test based on VO_2 max, or maximal oxygen uptake, a widely applied fitness standard. As the test beeps shorten and the speed gets faster minute by minute, more oxygen is needed to fuel the muscles. The lap count is ascribed a value—a predictor of maximal oxygen power, a student's fitness level. This is comparable to a treadmill test for adults.

Curiously, the use of Fitnessgram roughly parallels the increases in childhood obesity in America. How could that be? Meredith said it is "not an intervention, not a curriculum, not a program to improve fitness." It only *measures* fitness. And its guidelines only recommend testing once or twice a year because of the time involved in testing an entire student body with shrinking PE time.

With his monthly tests, which go on for a whole week, Dexter chooses to make Fitnessgram an intervention, a curriculum. He does the same with the mile runs, doing them twice a semester, four times a year, more than required. All running paths lead to the Healthy Kids Fun Run. Such nonstop reinforcement leads 9-year-old Alejandra, a fourth grader, to say after achieving a 40-lap personal best: "I practice every day. I run with my cousin. You get a lot of energy when you run against people."

HEALTHY STUDENTS KICK IT UP A NOTCH

Lynbrook's students bond and unite behind common goals. In the gym, the camaraderie is palpable. There's pride in learning, trust, a feeling that something important is being accomplished. McNamee, who came to Lynbrook four years ago, says the caring in the building is different from anything she's seen in her thirty years in education. She calls Dexter "Richard Dexter Disney Productions."

Dexter may be a Marine at heart, but he's no tin soldier. In front of the kids, he's equal parts Mick Jagger and Emeril Lagasse. "Every year, I try and kick it up a notch," he says.

At the Healthy Kids Fun Run, he sets up a postrace "base camp" with a banner, "Once a Leprechaun, Always a Leprechaun," as the kids groove to the music and float-size event mascots while glowing with runner's high. At the awards ceremony months later at a school assembly when event officials come with Marines and present a $500 check from its sponsor, the Washington-area *Family Magazine,* Dexter shines a spotlight on the kids and has smoke rise from a fog machine, like you see at pro sports events. At the Dream Mile on the school playground, Dexter choreographs a flag-raising ceremony and color guard and has the sixty-plus competitors (the youngest kids do a half mile) march to the start with Olympic-style pomp while he announces,

"The athletes are making their way up the field. . . . This is the Dream Mile!"

Dexter, who has a linebacker body, started running after college and went on to do four marathons with a best of 4:07. He felt his endomorph physique took too much of a beating, though, so he gave up running for swimming and now competes in masters swim events. He's still fit enough to log 74 laps—not quite as good as his best students—when he tries the Pacer Test himself.

In a third-grade class, 8-year-old Jason Truong runs as smoothly as any older kid I've seen, and should be ahead of the teacher before long. He works his way to 55 laps, a personal best by one lap. After getting a drink, he tells me, "I've been practicing all my life to become the best runner." His life began with kindergarten laps. He said that at the Healthy Kids Fun Run he was the first Lynbrook third grader across the finish line.

Not one second of the thirty-minute PE period is wasted. The class ends with mad sprinting to "Rock Around the Clock."

HEALTHY STUDENTS TEST THEIR SPEED

The youngest kids, kindergarten through second grades, enter the gym. They sprint "flat out," says Rich, despite his pacing pleas. "They're too young to go slow." For this group, he shortens the distance and does not record laps; the children are apprentices learning the ropes for third grade, when real testing begins. At the start, he has them "spread out like peanut butter." When the test gets under way, Rich runs a few laps with the kids to slow them down. "Watch me," he tells them. Still, even in street shoes, they dash ahead of him. Afterward, he discusses heart function and tells the kids to "walk after dinner with Mom and Dad."

Street shoes are not uncommon in Lynbrook's lineup at the Healthy Kids Fun Run, which is open to all youth 6 to 13. Dexter gets a kick out of seeing his kids outrunning well-off youngsters in fancy outfits. In a big change for 2008, Rick Nealis plans to add a fourth wave, for children and parents who want to run together. That should spike entries and help with safety.

With all its success, the Healthy Kids Fun Run has faced stumbling blocks. One year the "D.C. sniper" episode hurt entries. Another year, al-Qaeda threats reported in the newspapers hurt entries. At one time, the entry was free as long as a child came with a gift for the Marines' Toys for Tots program, but Nealis realized that many of these kids were the ones who should be *receiving* the toys. Then some schools could not afford to hire buses on the weekend. Now the race site is close to a D.C. Metro stop. As many as seventy Marines have been recruited to help manage the kids, but the numbers are down because of the war in Iraq.

Those who are able to help have a bit of pride to restore. A number of Marines choose to run with the fastest children, and it's not unheard of for a few soldiers to fade with fatigue. "One year they couldn't keep up with an 11-year-old," says Nealis. "Word spread at the base in Quantico." And then there was the time when it rained on race day and a high-ranking officer was summoned to instruct the field of young runners. When he spoke, there was no response. Just then, a child came out of the crowd, said something in Spanish, and the kids took off.

▶ Rules for Schools: Getting Students Running

1. **Facilities.** Modest facilities are not a deterrent because kids can run in any gym or playground.
2. **Time.** Limited PE class time is also not a deterrent because even weekly running can get kids started and enterprising teachers can develop additional running activities.
3. **Fun.** Running must always be framed as fun for kids, with motivations based on their age and background.
4. **Wellness.** Health issues can be introduced even to young

children, who can learn that feeling good, energetic, and calm is related to a vigorous, sweaty run.

5. Taboo. Never use running as punishment (such as giving children who misbehave extra laps).

6. Teachers. The most important factor in school-based running is an inspiring, dynamic teacher who earns the trust of students and parents while also generating administrative support.

7. Joy. Children of all ages and backgrounds have a natural joy in running that can be nurtured by caring educators.

8. Shoes. While children can run in ordinary clothing and sneakers they would use for other sports, parents should be encouraged to purchase running shoes to make running smoother and reduce risk of injury.

9. Aid. In communities in which families cannot afford running shoes, running stores (or the shoe companies themselves) can be approached for discounts or even complimentary gear, or schools can raise funds through bake sales and such.

10. Clubs. Local adult running clubs can provide mentors to help teachers develop programs, contribute hands-on coaching, educate parents, and offer children's fun runs and races.

11. Events. Many successful school programs are built around an out-of-school event that everyone can rally around—something teachers can use for extra motivation.

12. Expertise. PE teachers can enlist support from other teachers in the building with running experience.

13. Parents. Parent-runners can also play an important role in partnering with teachers and helping with after-school running.

14. Pride. School pride and a running identity are fostered with items kids can claim as their own, such as T-shirts, caps, and water bottles.

15. Mandates. PE teachers can use any required district or state physical fitness model to create a running program that more than meets minimum standards.

16. Enrichment. Any teacher can try to integrate running and other subject matter for cross-curriculum enrichment.

17. Structure. Create structured running routines that include warm-up exercises so that kids have expectations and responsibilities every time they run in class.

18. Records. Whether manually or in computer programs, keep records of students' running progress and give the kids a role in the recording process.

19. Rewards. Give kids modest rewards like buttons or patches for milestones such as miles or time run that they can wear proudly in school.

20. Bonding. Kids running in groups will develop camaraderie, supporting one another and reinforcing the joy of running.

21. Games. Whenever possible, running should be set up as games, relays, running to the start and stop of music, or a series of short runs, as opposed to continuous laps around the gym or field.

22. Pacing. Kids should learn how to pace themselves in order to sustain running for the duration of any instructional period.

23. Distance. With experience, growth, and fitness gains, youngsters should be able to cover between ½ to 2 miles of sustained running (about 5 to 20 minutes) comfortably.

24. Maturity. Running can be used to nurture students' ability to follow instructions, pay attention, delay gratification, set goals, and learn about their bodies.

25. Community. Teachers and parents can summon coaches of community sports teams to include running at practices and games.

26. After school. After-school running clubs are easy to organize with teachers and/or parents at the helm.

27. Families. Marathons and other races with corporate support have expanded into family-oriented events that are ideal for school participation.

28. Grants. Schools can apply for federal grants (such as from the Physical Education Program, or PEP) or private grants (such as those offered by the Robert Wood Johnson Foundation) to help fund running programs.

29. Dreams. A climactic school event with ceremonial color—like Lynbrook's Dream Mile—is an excellent driving force for schoolwide running, pride, and unity.

30. Standards. Hold students to high standards—not so much in pure performance but in trying hard and developing a sense of responsibility.

31. Themes. Create a theme that kids can understand and apply with all running—like Lynbrook's "personal best"— that serves as a cue for working hard and meeting goals.

32. Tradition. If you make running a school tradition, kids will look forward to running with little prodding and pass on the running attitude to each succeeding class.

5

Running with a Fast Pace

The key is learning to win, and lose, with grace and dignity, and to learn that every loss is an opportunity to get better.

—DR. BRENDA ARMSTRONG, COACH AND MEDICAL ADVISOR
OF THE DURHAM STRIDERS YOUTH TRACK SQUAD

*I*t is quite a sight: more than 100 youngsters ages 6 to 12 at a high school track in Durham, North Carolina, standing arm's length apart in rows of ten while doing stretching exercises in perfect unison. Well, almost perfect. When one boy misses a count in a set of jumping jacks, a volunteer coach, Darius Robinson, singles him out for criticism and orders the group to start over. Then the boy gets it right. The stretching continues with upward of a dozen exercises. Robinson barks instructions while using a hands-on approach to adjust kids' legs to the proper position: "Feet together! Lines straight!" The children quietly and crisply work their muscles and limbs in the second phase of their rigorous ninety-minute practice session at Hillside High School— they've already done a two-lap, half-mile warm-up—as they prepare for sprint work that will eventually lead them to championship youth track meets over the summer.

Tough love? You betcha.

The Durham Striders youth track and field team has been enforcing a zero-tolerance brand of discipline for thirty years now, and there's no room for softies with the spring track season under way. The team's godmother, Dr. Brenda Armstrong, one of the chief coaches and medical overseer, joins the crowd as additional adult reinforcement. She scrutinizes kids' stretching form, identifying the smallest imperfections, while Robinson reminds everyone that the team's first test of the season, an intrasquad meet on this same track, is only two days away. In gut-crunching abdominal work, he holds youngsters' raised legs low to the ground, to intensify the stomach stress, as kids let out a moan. "Take stretching seriously," he says. "No playing."

"This *is* tough love," Dr. Armstrong, a pediatric cardiologist and expert in youth running, tells me in an interview on the best ways to engage young runners in competition. "We yell and push the kids, but then we hug them. For many there are no hugs at home."

About 90 percent of the Durham Striders' 300 members (half of them are in middle school or high school and join team practices over the summer) are African American, most from low-income families, some new to the middle class. Dr. Armstrong says that before traveling to out-of-town meets many of the team members had never been out of Durham. The members of the Striders' community have overcome economic hardships to build a successful running program.

GIVING HUGS, REDUCING PRESSURE

Striders' hugs are not reserved for disadvantaged children. Dr. Armstrong points out one 10-year-old girl who attends private school, has been running with the Striders for three years, and excels in the 1,500 meters, and who will often come up to her saying, "I need a hug." It seems that the girl's father is pushing her to train more and more, beyond the three Striders practices a week—a serious breach of policy as far as Dr. Armstrong is concerned. The coaching staff insists that kids need to rest from the fairly intense Striders workouts and that additional running can be detrimental. "We've been doing this for many years," says the team co-founder and president, Frank Davis. "We know what works."

But the girl's father has his daughter running up to six days a week, as I find out myself when I speak to the girl later. Last summer, while still 9, she ran a 5:04 1,500 meters, one of the best in the country for her age and an excellent time for high school seniors twice her age. She says that in addition to Striders practices she trains up to three times a week with her dad; her workouts include hill repeats on a 300-meter incline and a long-distance run of 7 miles. When the Striders' season ends in August, instead of doing other sports like most of her teammates, the girl continues running year-round.

"I want to be a doctor and I want to go to the Olympics," she tells me.

With those goals at age 10, who wouldn't need a hug?

"She's feeling the pressure," says Dr. Armstrong. On a recent day she decided to confront the girl's father. "It came home to roost when she strained an Achilles tendon. I said to him in front of his daughter, 'Did she run over the weekend? I don't want her running fast at this time in the season.'"

With a team ethic that rallies youth to compete hard because "you have to compete in life" while defusing pushy parents who in effect co-opt their kids' athletic identity, Dr. Armstrong sits in the eye of the storm of youth sports and the debate over balancing high-profile achievement with more innocent goals of fun, fitness, and "letting kids be kids." And perhaps there's no single authority better equipped to weigh the issues than Dr. Armstrong. The daughter of a prominent coach who played many sports through school, Armstrong, 59, an associate professor of pediatrics at Duke University Medical Center and dean of admissions of Duke University Medical School, sees the effects of childhood obesity every day in her pediatric cardiology practice. As majordomo of the Durham Striders, she has helped nurture thousands of young runners in the last two decades and more.

The Durham approach, both in concept and in the alchemy of a team practice, provides a window into the methods that motivate and develop young runners who take up the call for competition. A child does not have to compete to experience the joy of running, make health gains, and learn strategies for the long-term. But racing adds an extra dimension with many additional benefits, and when competition is managed well as part of a team or club, a youngster's passion for running can be boundless.

RUNNING KIDS CAN HAVE IT ALL

As Dr. Armstrong sees it, a child can have it all. He or she can train hard but feel eager, learn how to win *and* lose, and gain toughness on the track and sensitivity off it. With Durham's values-based approach, in which good citizenship is prized and report cards are checked, plus its relentless emphasis on family nutrition, youngsters are embraced by a full-scale health assault in which bad habits are corrected, new ideas emerge, and the team serves as a society unto itself. If it takes a village to raise a child, the Durham Striders are as good as any.

The proof is not only in the statistics—which show numerous individual and team championships in youth events, over 200 college scholarships earned, and many adult track stars among the alumni—but also in the maturity of these young runners, who see hard work as a privilege, rise to leadership roles, and try their best to drink the required 64 ounces of water per day. The proof is in the way educators such as Dr. Armstrong and the other coaches, all volunteers, can shrink the presumed chasm between running to win and running for fun so that both ideas coexist in a motif that could be called "healthy intensity."

Running track is a culture unto itself, even for kids. Compared with road racing or cross-country, a track race leaves little room for error or lapse in focus. Confidence is not an option. Run every race as a fighter; shake hands afterward. And so last year's new Durham T-shirt with "No Mercy" inscribed on the back has been a big hit with the kids, who earn the shirts with race efforts and strong practices. The message is, never show mercy to your competition or to yourself in giving in to weakness. When I tell Dr. Armstrong that the idea could be construed as pretty hard-core, she refers to another youth team in the area that, she says, conveys to the children that it doesn't matter whether they win or lose. "The problem with that," she says, "is that life is about competition. It is unrealistic to think that children will not learn that quickly, before they're 5 years old. The key is learning to win, and lose, with grace and dignity, and to learn that every loss is an opportunity to get better."

Team parents echo that view. Anita Hunt, an attorney with four youngsters on the team, tells me at practice that the phrase "doesn't mean we are not kind-hearted. It means we are out here as a team, as a family, to do our best."

TEAM SUPPORT AND MOTIVATION

All of the burgeoning competitive opportunities for youth—whether in track, cross-country, or family fun runs—are enhanced by having the family atmosphere and support of a team or club. No one type of group, coach, training system, or competitive emphasis is right for every child or family. Perhaps the greatest benefit of most teams is giving youngsters a separate sphere of influence from parents, to minimize the chances of kids doing too much for their age, assuming that the coach has the knowledge and understanding to guide youngsters properly. Sharing in running and racing with peers also takes the edge off, keeping it fun even while goals are sought and training is intensified.

Few youth teams have the benefit of a physician (a pediatric cardiologist yet) on call and helping at practices; in that regard, Durham may be unique. Dr. Armstrong monitors team members' blood pressure, finding initial hypertension levels reduced to healthy readings—as a result of exercise and improved nutrition—in the course of a track season. She also finds reduced body fat and improved heart functioning. Children with resting pulse rates of 90 to 100 beats per minute at the start of practice have heart-healthy measures of about 70 by season's end. The coaches see a correlation between improved fitness and better grades and behavior.

COMPETING IN A HEALTHY MANNER

For children to compete in a healthy manner consistent with age, temperament, and goals, consider the following guidelines, some recommended by Dr. Armstrong and the Durham Striders.

EVENTS AND SEASONS

As with older runners, children and preteens have cross-country meets in the fall, indoor track events in winter, outdoor track events in spring and summer, and road races year-round. Cross-country has special appeal with large fields running on winding, hilly park trails, at times in muddy conditions. It features a free-form atmosphere kids thrive on. Youth cross-country leagues offering a series of races with team and individual scoring are found all around the country and can be checked out on the Web. The

strength building that's a part of cross-country also provides an
excellent foundation for track or road racing later on. In the winter, there are indoor meets here and there for youth. The venera-
ble Colgate Women's Games, now in its thirty-third year, is a big
draw in the New York City area, with girls' events starting in first
grade and qualifying rounds leading to a final in Madison Square
Garden. Spring and summer track opportunities are abundant.
National programs with regional meets include USA Track and
Field Junior Olympics and Youth Championships and Hershey's
Track and Field Games (see the appendix for event listings).

AGE AND DISTANCE

A hallmark of the Durham program is playing to children's
strengths. They keep distances short, which appeals to youngsters' short attention spans and avoids taxing young bodies with
too much pounding. Plus, a child's instinct is to run short and
fast. Miles can be added later, as the youngster grows. For kids 5
to 8, Dr. Armstrong recommends events up to a half mile or
maybe a mile, tops; for those 9 to 12, events up to 3,000 meters
(1.8 miles) or 2 miles. She says studies have shown that too much
running prior to adolescence puts undue wear and tear on the
growth plates. Therefore, she's not a fan of 5K (3.1 miles) racing
for preteens but feels it's acceptable as long as it's infrequent and
done for pure fun and not time goals. Better yet, she says, if a
child runs with one or both parents, the child's focus will be on
the parent as opposed to a performance standard. The longest Junior Olympics event in the 11–12 division is 1,500 meters (just
short of a mile). Most children's events at road races and marathons are a mile and under. The excellent Girls on the Run program centers on 5K events but the training is low-key and goals
revolve around values and self-esteem.

JOINING A TEAM OR CLUB

Check the Web for local teams and use word of mouth and the running community network for advice. Running stores, adult clubs, road races, health clubs, sports medicine facilities, school teams, and coaches are among the best sources. Find out about a team's training methods and facilities, competitive emphasis, size of squad and age group, expectations, costs and—most important—who's in charge. Dr. Armstrong suggests that a team that does not have a preseason orientation to review its approach and answer questions is one to avoid. Coaches differ widely, from those keyed on a trophy collection to others, like Armstrong, who focus on a holistic, child-centered approach. Security is critical. How is practice supervised? Is the facility (track, park, gym) safe? Are kids running out on the road in traffic? Be sure at least one adult remains at practice until the last child is picked up.

IF THE SHOE FITS

At the Durham practice, the youngsters wear all manner of clothing, some geared for running, some not. But every child has regulation running shoes, which Dr. Armstrong, as a physician, is adamant about. She says, "Between 6 and 12, a child's feet are not growing at the same pace; one foot is bigger than the other. The same is true with the legs. At 11 or 12, some youngsters have Osgood Schlatters [knee pain during growth spurt, affecting more boys than girls]. They are prone to shin splints and ankle instability. They must be put in shoes that help their running, not work against them." Most reputable running specialty stores will be helpful but make sure they carry kids' sizes. (For more on kids' running shoes, see chapter 2.)

POSITIVE PEER PRESSURE

Kids on a running team acquire immediate role models in a positive environment. Unlike other sports in which being a starter, amount of playing time or points scored creates a pressure-packed caste system that turns many kids off, young runners see older kids doing stretching exercises, enjoying running, working hard and spreading goodwill among all team members. Kids pick up on the "rightness" of the endeavor. They don't compete against teammates but *with* them for the greater good of the group. Before long, the youngsters become role models themselves.

COMPETITIVE SPIRIT

Youngsters vary in their comfort level with competition. Some children may love the camaraderie and friendships of a team without being fixed on the racing itself. The more competitive youngsters, says Dr. Armstrong, are very attentive to coaches, are not easily distracted, and even approach the coaches with questions about doing better. Another benefit of a team is helping parents determine what their kids really want out of running. Oftentimes, reluctant competitors without a team may run races to go along with parents' wishes, but in a team setting coaches can objectively assess kids and inform parents. Conversely, children shy about racing when pushed by parents may warm to competition with the support of peers, newfound knowledge, and other team-oriented features.

TRAINING PERIODS

Durham's program runs from March into August, five months. In 2008, Dr. Armstrong added optional winter conditioning once a week, on Saturdays; many parents turned out to train with their kids, and some youngsters did a couple of low-key indoor track races. A five- or six-month running period is plenty for kids as long as they are active the rest of the year. After track, most of the Durham kids play football, basketball, soccer, or tennis; some, after a running break, do a little cross-country. A child should not be encouraged to specialize in running year-round. If they do, they increase their risk of burnout and injury. Most of the nation's marathon-connected kids' programs are three-to-six-month incremental buildups. Girls on the Run uses a twelve-week plan twice a year.

TRAINING APPROACHES

Easy jogging a few days a week will help kids get in shape for racing, but for competitive advantage more speed and structure are advised. Durham's training is based on fast laps of the track. The 5-to-8 group will run eight 300s in two sets of four. They take a complete rest between runs, starting with 8 minutes of rest and working down to 2 minutes through the season. A 10-minute rest between sets is gradually reduced to 5 minutes. Likewise, the 9-to-12 group will run eight 400s in two sets of four, with a similar rest pattern as the younger kids. Durham coaches say they "work from a 400-meter base," meaning that 400s give youngsters both the speed and strength to compete in any event from 100 meters to 1,500 meters.

STRESSING YOUNG BODIES

Dr. Armstrong checks kids' breathing to make sure they're not overtaxed. "I can tell not only how fast they're breathing but how deeply they're breathing," she says. Experienced coaches can do the same. At the practice I witness, most of the team does a series of repeat 150s. I also see a lot of limbering up. The key to avoiding fatigue is the three-day-a-week regimen. A 10-year-old Durham youngster might log three miles (including warm-up) per practice, less than 10 miles a week. This is easier on a child's growing body than jogging 3 or 4 miles a day six or seven days a week (especially year-round). It's also easier on the mind. Tell a youngster to go run 3 miles (about 30 minutes) and he might find that boring and probably not look forward to it the next time.

PACING PRIORITIES

Kids, at first, know two speeds: fast and slow. There's a range of middle speeds to be learned. Without teammates and coaching, most youngsters will only run slowly in a jogging manner, missing out on the intricacies of running and variation of experience. With more "running sense," kids will more readily find a running groove, tire less, learn to compete, and set the stage for future growth.

PRACTICE PARTS

Any practice, whether as fine-tuned as Durham's, or not should have (1) a jogging warm-up, (2) stretching, (3) drills and stride-outs (several short, fast runs of about 50 meters at less than full speed), (4) the main part of workout with distance and/or sprints, (5) cool-down jogging, and (6) final stretching. Durham kids jog two laps, 800 meters (about a half mile), when they arrive at the track. Stretching is vigorous, working all parts of the body (see sidebar). Then they line up for quick 50-meter runs plus drills such as high knees, skipping, and butt kicks (accentuating leg action so the feet just about touch the rear end as they run). They do another easy lap before the heart of their workout: the sprint repeats. They finish with another easy lap and more stretching. Girls and boys do the same.

▶ Stretch Like the Striders: Loosey-Goosey in Durham

After a youngster jogs about 5 minutes to warm up the body and stimulate blood flow, he or she can follow this stretching routine of fourteen exercises done by the Durham Striders track squad. (For additional stretches, see chapter 2, page 48.)

Jumping jacks. Do 25 full jumping jacks, bringing hands together above head. *Benefits:* whole body.

Toe touches. Keeping knees straight, bend slowly, and try to touch toes. Hold for a count of 5 and repeat three times. *Benefits:* hamstring muscles, lower back.

Head bends. Keeping knees straight, bend to one side, and grab ankle with both hands, pulling head to knee. Hold for a count of 5 and repeat three times, trying to get head closer each time. Do both sides. *Benefits:* hamstring muscles.

Crossovers. Stand with right foot over left foot and, keeping knees straight, try to touch toes. Hold for a count of 5 and repeat three times. Do both sides. *Benefits:* hamstring muscles.

Foot grab. With feet shoulder width apart and pointed straight, keeping knees straight, bend to one side and use both hands to try and touch foot. Hold for a count of 5 and repeat three times. Do both sides. *Benefits:* hamstring muscles.

Butt reach. With feet spread wider than shoulder width, bend from the torso, keeping knees straight, and put hands underneath the body to reach butt. Hold for 10 seconds and repeat once. *Benefits:* hamstring muscles.

Groin stretch. With right foot in front of body and left foot back, keeping feet straight, knees bent and hands on opposite sides of front foot, lead forward with your head. Hold for a count of 5. Do both sides. *Benefits:* groin and calf muscles and hips.

Forward lean. Seated on the ground with legs together, toes pointing up and knees straight, lean from the torso and try to touch toes. Hold for 10 seconds. *Benefits:* hamstring muscles.

Seated head bend. Seated on the ground with legs spread wide and knees straight, bend head toward the knee. Hold for 5 seconds and repeat. Do both sides. *Benefits:* hamstring muscles.

Seated groin stretch. Seated on the ground with legs spread wide and knees straight, lean forward, bringing your head to the ground. Hold for 10 seconds. *Benefits:* groin muscles.

Backward lean. Seated on the ground with left leg forward and right leg bent back so it is about at a right angle to the left leg, bring torso backward toward the ground. Hold for count of 5 and repeat. Do both sides. *Benefits:* back and quadriceps muscles.

Leg lifts. Lie on your back, keeping legs together, and raise both legs about a foot off the ground. Hold for 10 seconds and repeat five times. *Benefits:* abdominal and quadriceps muscles.

Chest raise. Lie on stomach and lift chest with hands out front and legs extended back. Hold for 10 seconds and repeat. *Benefits:* abdominal muscles.

Sit-ups. Lie on back with legs bent and hands together at chest and bring head to knees. Repeat for as long as 60 seconds while maintaining form. *Benefits:* abdominal muscles.

GROWTH AND MATURITY

Grooming kids to race is equal parts art and science. The art is to know how children differ and make adjustments to address those differences. Kids grow and mature at different rates. They learn in different ways: some by listening, some by watching, others by doing. A struggling 8-year-old may become a successful 10-year-old. Be patient and flexible. There is no deadline for a child to achieve. To spice up the menu, coaches give kids hills to run; they enjoy going up and down, and hills tend to improve form because you can't run a hill with bad form (like leaning backward). On the track, a child having trouble completing laps can just run the turns, then jog the straightaway, turn around, and repeat. Do whatever keeps him or her moving and interested, such as trying new distances. Avoid running the same race over and over. Discipline should vary too. As Frank Davis says, "Some kids you can 'yell' at. Others you can't—they just cry right away."

A RELAY GOOD IDEA

At practice and meets, put kids on relays. Place a baton in a child's hand and watch him fly! Baton-passing skills require finesse and offer a great learning opportunity. Relay events for youth are usually 4 × 100, 4 × 200, or 4 × 400, so they're getting sprint work, running fast, and learning to function as part of a group. It's a win-win situation. On a winning team all four members (even the slowest) are winners; on a team that does not do that well, no one child is at fault (except in a baton-passing mishap or rules violation). Relays provide excitement and drama. There's no pressure and a barrel of fun. A child running a number of relays in practice does what amounts to a whole workout without realizing it, gaining confidence for individual racing.

GOOD GRADES

Dr. Armstrong believes that many schools today have practically given up on their role in teaching discipline, character and values, and taking responsibility for one's actions. The Striders attempt to fill that gap with a code of conduct that kids and parents must sign. Vulgar language, fighting, disrespect toward coaches, and other undesirable behavior are not tolerated and can be grounds for expulsion. Durham seeks to produce not only good runners but productive citizens. Report cards are checked, and if grades are not up to speed youngsters are disallowed from practice for a couple of weeks to work harder on homework and such. Everything Durham does—and it's what running should essentially be about for all families—is to empower youngsters to lead healthy lives.

HEALTHY EATING

At Durham, empowerment is most emphatic when it comes to diet, a sore spot with Dr. Armstrong. She sees the devastating impact of poor diet in her patient care. Team rules include no soda, potato chips, processed meats, bacon, or hot dogs ("like pouring a salt shaker down your throat"). Armstrong urges parents to have something nutritious ready for kids when they get home from school. Her list includes fresh veggies like carrots or broccoli, trail mix, or peanut butter and jelly on whole grain bread. For drinks, only water. "When you sweat, you lose water," she says. For kids to comply, many families have to make fundamental changes in how they eat. Armstrong checks on compliance weekly and asks kids to remind parents of healthy food choices.

HANDLING HEAT

To keep kids healthy and hydrated for running, Dr. Armstrong has a 64-ounce (8 glasses) rule for daily water intake, and even more on really hot days. That may be an ambitious goal but at least drinking will be a constant. In the summer, water bottles should be kept in the freezer overnight so they will still be cold at the next day's practice. At practice, Dr. Armstrong has no problem telling the assemblage, "The way to know if you're drinking enough is, if your pee is yellow you're not drinking enough water. It should be clear."

PARENTS' BOTTOM LINE

For kids' racing, Dr. Armstrong offers a three-pronged bottom line:

1. "Let the kids have fun," she says. "When you apply hardcore competitive approaches to a young child, there's a predictable end. If you push too hard, at some point the child will burn out. They cannot be treated like a Thoroughbred horse."
2. Dr. Armstrong points out that, "as opposed to teenagers and adults, the children you're dealing with are people whose bodies are changing. Children may do better at different distances depending on their development. Let them make their own choices at each stage of growth."
3. "Children have to develop an identity of their own, not one of their parents," she reminds parents. I have one kid whose dad is always on me because he was a sprinter and he wants his son to be a sprinter. The boy prefers longer distance like the 800. I tell the father, 'What did your son tell you today? What is more important—your ego or his happiness?'"

At times, Armstrong finds a diplomatic solution that satisfies everyone. She convinced the boy to run sprints on a relay, which he enjoyed. And to nurture his independence, she started calling him "Superman," giving him an identity he liked. When he arrives at the track, Armstrong calls out, "How's Superman doing today?"

▶ Durham Striders Parent: 4 Runners 4 Discipline

Anita Hunt, a 42-year-old attorney who ran for the Durham Striders herself in the club's early days, has four children currently in the program: Tre (14), Lauren (10), Nigel (9), and Ryan (7). Here's what she likes about Durham's approach to running, health, and character building.

Training and racing. "There's nothing easy about running track, no matter what the event. It takes perseverance and resiliency. Sometimes it hurts but you still finish the race. Those are life lessons."

Nutrition. "We had to cut down on fried foods and make a huge increase in water intake. We also have a drink called 'Naked' that combines fruits, vegetables, vitamins, and minerals. These are lifestyle changes that will benefit my children in the long-term."

Health. "When the kids take their annual physicals, the pediatrician sees their healthy hearts and other evidence of physical fitness. I know that running helps with hypertension, especially in the African American community, and with cholesterol issues."

Report card standards. "I love it. It's a fantastic incentive to do well on and off the track."

Role model. "For the Saturday gym workouts in the winter, Dr. Armstrong allowed parents to participate. I worked out with my kids and since then I've lost 21 pounds."

▶ Anita Hunt's Son Nigel, a 9-Year-Old Third Grader, Talks About His Running

Q: How many years are you running for Durham?

Nigel: This is my fourth year.

Q: What are your events and times?

Nigel: Last summer I ran 5:11 in the 1,500 and won a gold medal in the Junior Olympics. I also ran 2:37 in the 800 and 67 in the 400.

Q: What do you like most about running?

Nigel: The medals and trophies.

Q: What's your favorite kind of practice?

Nigel: 300s.

Q: Why?

Nigel: Because they're short.

Q: What other sports do you do?

Nigel: Basketball and soccer.

Q: What's your favorite subject in school?

Nigel: PE.

Q: Can you describe how you feel when you run?

Nigel: No.

Q: What's your diet like?

Nigel: I eat cereal for breakfast and lunch.

Q: Why would you tell a runner to join Durham?

Nigel: They're better than other track teams.

▶ Racing Routines: Eat, Drink, Stay Cool, Run Fast

Dr. Armstrong's tips for race readiness:

The night before: Have pasta and salad for dinner.

Breakfast day of race: Have whole-wheat pancakes or waffles with syrup at least three hours before the race. No milk or milk products, orange juice with pulp, margarine, sausage, or bacon.

Drinking: Have at least 32 ounces of water prior to the race.

Heat: On hot days, before the race stay in the shade as much as possible, even while warming up. Dress in light colors and loose-fitting clothes. Wear a cap.

Warm-ups: About an hour before the race, do easy jogging, stretches, and some wind sprints. If you're on a team, listen to team leaders or captains. Sip water.

Smart racing: Report on time to the start, listen to officials' instructions, be confident and relaxed, and pace yourself properly. Remember that you're in excellent shape from all your practices.

Postrace snack: Have trail mix or peanut butter and jelly on wheat bread. Sip water.

▶ Relax, and Run Your Best: *Smart Sports Psyching*

Philadelphia sports psychologist Joel Fish, Ph.D., who counsels young athletes as well as professionals, offers the following advice on competition for children and teens in his excellent book *101 Ways to Be a Terrific Sports Parent* (Fireside/Simon & Schuster), co-written with Susan Magee:

- **Prerace jitters**—like dry mouth and sweaty palms—are normal and can actually help performance.
- **Parents should** adopt a calm demeanor because excessive stress in adults will make children that much more anxious.
- **Reciting a** mantra like "Just do your best" or "I am a winner" can serve as positive cues for youngsters.
- **Practice deep** breathing to relieve undue stress. Breathe deeply through the nose while pushing the stomach out.

Let your chest fill with air. Hold for a count of 4. Then exhale slowly to a count of 8. Repeat as needed. Think of it as exhaling the tension out of your body.

- **Use children's** performance, whether successful or not, as a learning experience for future efforts.

6

Running with "Practice Phobia"

When you're on a team it's like family. Running is about a group of people working and striving to reach the next goals.

—SASHA ESTRELLA-JONES, SEVENTH-GRADE RUNNER
AT A BROOKLYN, NEW YORK, MIDDLE SCHOOL

If you ask a 13-year-old a question, especially a 13-year-old runner, brace yourself—you can never be sure what you'll find out. One fine spring day at Leif Erickson Park in the Bay Ridge section of Brooklyn, at the Intermediate School 30 Young Runners team practice, I ask 13-year-old Sasha Estrella-Jones what she likes about running.

"When I'm running," she says, "it's like an obstacle and I just want to break the wall down and push so hard so I can get to the next level and I'm even better and have more challenges. Because when I have a challenge in front of me—which is what running for me is all about—it pushes me to be better. And I make lots of friends on this team and it's also really healthy for me, especially since I have asthma, it helps me so much in my running."

This young lady is a seventh grader. She is in her second year of running and can race 4 miles in just under 35 minutes, about 8:44 per mile. As she speaks, Estrella grows even more passionate and convincing, raising her voice and gesturing like a church preacher, and I take advantage of the moment, asking what she's learned from the coach and how she motivates herself.

"The coach is all about team," Estrella tells me. "We rise and fall together. I really like that because she taught me that teamwork is something bigger than yourself. When you're on a team, it's like family. Running is about a group of people working and striving to reach the next goals."

Estrella is on break between sprints as the rest of her squad, thirty strong, boys and girls ages 11 to 14 in the sixth, seventh, and eighth grades, are sent off on park loops by head coach Calliope (Callie) Anthanasakos, whom the kids call Miss A. They have a track meet coming up—a youth jamboree conducted by the New York Road Runners Foundation—at Icahn Stadium on Randall's Island, and Callie supervises a tune-up workout of 4 × 100, 3 × 200, and 2 × 400, with plenty of stretching exercises.

There's no stopping Estrella, on or off the track. She continues, "Some days you're feeling down and your teammates try to bring you up. It comes to a point, if I want people to help me, I have to help myself. It's that light inside of you that triggers all, and you have to hit that mark and keep going and show what you got inside of you."

With both sprints and distance on Estrella's menu, I can't resist one last question—does she prefer the sprints or adult-level Central Park road races? "Short distance I understand and like. But in long distance that endurance just kicks in and adrenaline pumps. When I'm out there running with adults I get the vibe the adults give the kids. I feel, this is for me, this is for my team, and I just have to push."

"PRACTICE PHOBIA" BUILDS CONFIDENCE

Pushing the body at a hard pace can intimidate a 13-year-old who is not as secure as Estrella, as I found out the day before my IS 30 visit while attending a New York City middle school association track meet at Icahn Stadium. This time, my Gen R (for running) spokesperson is a boy, Chi Yang Cheng, an eighth grader at Hunter College Middle School in Manhattan, who recently asked his coach, Tiffanie Clarke, "Is it possible for me to have 'practice phobia'?"

Practice *what*? Chen, who lives in Forest Hills, Queens, takes two subway lines to school, and lets his hair cover his face, explains. "Where we run in Central Park, it's pretty hard for me. I remember it as unpleasant when we practiced for cross-country." The spot of intimidation is the notorious 110th Street hill on the park's north end. "Sometimes I like to go crazy to calm myself down. I know it sounds weird. Going crazy calms me. Like . . ." Chi demonstrates with a scream and broad gestures, "Arghhh-hhh!" and says that as "reverse" therapy he tells himself, "I'm sooo scared!" Clearly, he's sports psychologist material. "It relaxes me. It helps me realize the hill is not as hard as I think it is. After going crazy, I calm down and tell myself, 'I have practice phobia.' That mellows me out."

This is New York, baby, where newly minted teens are hip and hyped and, I'm finding out, running a lot stronger and smarter than even I would have imagined. As the IS 30 sign in the lobby announces: this is "where wildcats roar." That would seem a bold posture for a tiny school (by New York standards) whose 340 students don't even have a regulation school building but a converted three-story apartment house with no gym. PE classes are held in the music room. For the space to run in fitness testing, the student body had to be shipped to another school.

"We're so small there's no escaping," Elizabeth Maley, the assistant principal, tells me. "We know all the kids. There are friendships among sixth, seventh, and eighth graders. I have not seen this in other schools." This camaraderie is all the more impressive as the population is a mix of many religions and ethnic backgrounds. Ten-year-old IS 30, also called the Mary White Ovington School, is a Title I school with at least 60 percent of families below the federal poverty level.

While urban middle schools can be boisterous and unruly, Ovington is a model of decorum, led by the running team, which comprises almost 10 percent of all students. The runners' maturity, says Maley, the after-school supervisor, sets an example. "Putting yourself out there in weekend meets requires a lot of self-confidence, which is lacking at this age," she says. "If you can develop that in the early teen years, it's very significant."

And this stretch of Brooklyn, though situated at the four-mile point of the New York City Marathon, is hardly running country. There's no greenery with sweeping meadows or leg-friendly dirt trails. The nearest track is a drive away at Fort Hamilton High (where 1976 Olympic decathlete Fred Samara got his start), and the nearest park, Leif Erickson, is a concrete maze that was 40 percent deforested when a freak tornado with winds up to 135 mph swept through the neighborhood last year.

"GUERRILLA RUNNING" YIELDS URBAN LEGENDS

"We call it 'guerrilla running,'" says Cliff Sperber, executive director of the New York Road Runners Foundation, of how most city running teams scrape by. It was the foundation's school program that paved the way for the IS 30 running team. The Young Runners division, oriented toward middle schools, has grown to 64 school teams and 2,500 youngsters throughout the five boroughs. A few schools have over 100 team members. (There's also an elementary school division, Mighty Milers, serving over 50,000 children, and a City Sports for Kids track program.) The

Foundation provides training seminars for interested Young Runners coaches, athlete incentives like T-shirts for attending practices, free entries into club-sponsored track, cross-country, and road racing events, and even bus transportation to meets. "The whole program is free to the kids," says Young Runners program manager Paola Baptiste. The club recommends that teams practice at least twice a week for an hour or more and provides a training CD with an array of workouts. Competition ranges from 100 meters to the 10K.

The only cost is a coach's after-hours stipend paid by the school. Even this minor amount becomes an issue. Because of Board of Education budget cuts, Callie's twice-weekly two-hour practices have been reduced to a rushed 90 minutes. Her system: leave school at 3:00, walk with a band of thirty-plus youngsters through traffic to the park, get there at 3:15, practice for an hour, walk back as a group, and clock in at 4:30 sharp so parents can pick up kids and the security cop can leave. That requires coaching precision and extraordinary "classroom" management.

Callie and her staff—assistant coach Liza Schneider (a science teacher) and parent volunteer Tammy Castellanos (whose son was in the program)—make it work. With this typically difficult age group, such discipline is easily taken for granted. In fact, Baptiste, who has joined me in the visit, says that at some schools where coaches do not have adequate control of their student-runners, a foundation field manager is sent to help "refocus practice."

At IS 30, the NYRR field manager is needed only to run with the stronger youngsters so they can venture to the Verrazano Bridge and back, 6 miles. Callie says the off-site effort gives her lesser runners a chance to shine at practice and boost their self-esteem. You can't talk about this delicate age group without emphasizing self-esteem.

The 6-miler is crucial in offering the type of challenge Estrella talks about. Otherwise, distance runs are done Brooklyn-style, around the block, with Callie, Liz, and Tammy positioned on three corners to monitor the kids and make sure that taunts from those at other schools ("IS 30 sucks") are held at bay. It is two and a half laps per mile, says Callie, and so the team's 4-milers work out to 10 laps of a full city block.

Team member Jalal Alassari, a 13-year-old seventh grader, tells me his favorite run so far is the Verrazano 6-miler. He says he's done it without stopping in 52 minutes. And, without being asked, Jalal offers, "I felt proud of myself."

How anyone can inspire kids this age—with their hormones, peer pressure, and the nonstop distractions of being a kid in the world today—to look forward to running several miles around the block or through the streets after school is why I have returned to my New York roots. I want to see it for myself. I grew up in Brooklyn, ran high school meets at Randall's Island, and once taught in a New York City junior high.

My high school had no track either and in the winter we ran the school hallways. IS 30's hallways are too short for running, so in winter the team spreads out over all three floors for stretching and strengthening exercises. It takes pretty bad weather to force the Wildcats indoors. Callie says that initially she had parents complaining when the kids ran in the rain or cold. She's had to educate parents as well as children.

INSPIRED IN CITY, SUBURB, AND ELITE ZIP CODES

It's clear that people, not perks, make for successful young runners. Bay Ridge may be gritty, but it also has a comforting neighborhood feel. The sidewalks around IS 30 feature restaurants with a dozen ethnic cuisines; Islamic and pan-Hellenic cultural centers; Methodist, Lutheran, and Catholic churches; Archie Bunker row houses; and the Jerusalem Barber Shop, $8 a cut. There is not a Starbucks in sight.

In urban areas, kids and coaches learn to tough it out. Maybe that's okay for middle schoolers, who are trying to transition from coddled children to more independent young people. Many frustrated educators have thrown up their hands over this group, uncertain whether the old model of the middle school years still warrants its own turf. Should school pathways be kindergarten through eighth grade, then high school? If we have middle schools, should they be grades five through seven, six through eight, or seven through nine?

Regardless of how they're categorized, these tweens may offer the best raw material for running. They're old enough to form opinions, and while many think they know it all, that's just emotional cover for being, in the vernacular, clueless. As they prepare for the next stage of life as fully realized teenagers—possibly as high school runners—they desperately need adult guidance. And many are getting it. I find that from IS 30 to the city's private schools ranks to my own New Jersey suburbs, middle school coaching, while often taking a bad rap, has some of the most thoughtful and dedicated people in the business.

Many coaches learn that running offers salvation to young teens increasingly stressed by family and cultural issues. A 2000 study published in the *Journal of Personality and Social Psychology* found that normal children 9 to 17 were more anxious than children treated for psychiatric disorders fifty years ago. One reason, according to the research, was physical isolation, affected by high divorce rates and less community involvement, among other factors. What better response could there be than a close-knit running team where kids are nurtured and challenged but, at the same time, not judged?

At IS 30, coach Anthanasakos, 33, an English teacher and occasional runner reared on church basketball leagues, says, "I believe I'm teaching a life philosophy. It's not English or track but creating a foundation for the students to build upon and become successful adults. I want children to challenge themselves, to encourage one another, to forge strong bonds."

That Socratic approach has a long tradition at St. Benedict's, a 104-year-old boys' K-8 private school in Manhattan, where head track coach Eric Hill, who handles fifth through eighth graders, says, "Our running program offers a place for the more unique students in the school. They are not necessarily the kind of guys who would play baseball or lacrosse. They're sort of eccentric, a bright group. It has spread around school that you can run, get in shape, and have a good time."

In the suburbs, eccentricity is not easily rewarded, and at Marlboro Middle School in Monmouth County, New Jersey, boys cross-country and girls track coach Caolan Sinisi, a special ed teacher, plays with convention like a sculptor working the edges of the human form. She says, "People say I'm crazy for coaching middle school: the hormones, the attitudes, especially the 'I'm too cool' attitude. I suppose I am a little crazy because these things that others complain about are what I love about these evolutionary creatures we call middle schoolers. They thrive on discipline, prosper on order, and flourish on schedules. Track and cross-country are so important for them."

20 RULES FOR MIDDLE SCHOOLS

Here is what we have learned so far about creating a positive running environment for the middle school age group:

1. They are smarter and more sensitive than we might realize and appreciate the challenges put before them.
2. They thrive on teamwork and sharing the running experience with peers.
3. They are mature enough to make group goals a priority

and understand that group success will lead to personal success.

4. Boys and girls can work together and learn to respect one another as equals.

5. Kids of different ages can support one another and learn to respect different ability levels.

6. Some kids fear hard training and need extra time in adapting to physical stress.

7. They can excel at many distances and are best served by sampling a variety of events.

8. They can be trained to run long distances and race in 5K and 10K events.

9. They can excel regardless of family background and income level.

10. They can always use a boost in self-confidence and self-esteem.

11. They like to be organized and do things according to regular schedules.

12. They can train anywhere as long as the environment is safe.

13. Smart, strong coaching is crucial in providing leadership and motivation.

14. Coaching attitudes and passion are more important than training expertise.

15. External rewards—incentives—are fine enhancements as long as kids learn to enjoy running from within.

16. Adult running clubs are usually willing to lend a hand with organizational help, training ideas, and events to run.

17. Parent volunteers are important in providing additional supervision and as liaison with all the youngsters' moms and dads.

18. They can run in inclement weather but in extreme condi-

tions should use indoor facilities for alternative conditioning.
19. Despite their protests, they are comfortable with discipline as long as policies are flexible and fair.
20. When integrated into the educational process with com-
munal values, running can enhance the middle school
runner's total well-being.

Getting middle school kids to make a commitment to running requires a delicate balance of competitive fire and a non-
threatening atmosphere, what coach Eric Hill calls "excessive
moderation." He says, "They're growing and there are sinews
and ligaments and muscles to protect. You don't want to scare
them off."

It's probably the psyche that needs protecting most. Hill, a
PE teacher at St. Bernard's who has also taught English and history, takes a laid-back approach, letting youngsters choose their
events and define success on their own terms. As a New York
City Marathon participant, he's a good role model, and even at
56 he can join in the team fun, the inside jokes, "our little world"
that distinguishes runners and gives them a sense of independence.

Hill is so laid-back that when a youngster who is the grandson
of a former world record holder said he was thinking of coming
out for track, Hill told him, "Sure, if that's what you want to do."
Then, after running down the hall in private jubilation, Hill told
the boy later on, "I know that in your family track can be a sensitive issue. I'm not concerned about your grandfather. He's not
running. You are."

But Hill gets results. St. Bernard's has some of the best sprint-
ers in the middle school league. And his fifth and sixth graders
are showing distance promise, with big improvements from training in Central Park. In less than a year, they've improved from 19

minutes to 14 minutes for a 1.6-mile route. Their training is a mere 2 miles a day four days a week; Hill's older runners do about twice that.

At the Icahn competition where I meet Hill, his less-is-more ethos is mirrored by many other private school coaches, and the athletes reflect that, showing a grace and humility that belies their reputation as spoiled rich kids. On a cold, windswept day, as parents huddle in blankets, some youngsters compete in sweatsuits and sneakers, those doing the hurdles barrel across the line laughing, and no one seems to get upset when one 200-meter runner stops before the finish line. The aura of play is everywhere.

This same track, which hosts the world-class Reebok International every year and is as fine a facility as any after a $10 million makeover courtesy of financier Carl Icahn, sees girls of all shapes and sizes from schools like Dalton, Spence, and Dwight line up for the 800 meters, won in 2:42, a good time but not headline material. The winner wears some protective device on both knees. She says that her hips are wide and inflexible (typical of girls this age) and the coverings prevent her knees from knocking together.

COOL KIDS WITH SMART IDEAS

These are cool kids, not because of elitism but because running has given them direction and maturity. Celina Dubin, a Spence seventh grader, is happy with her third-place finish in the 800 and also happy about her decision to do many sports and not specialize in tennis, in which she excels, year-round. She says that each sport complements the others and that she is learning to run distance events, a step up from her initial sprinting. Her mother, Eva, notes that her daughter's busy schedule (travel team soccer, basketball, etc.) makes her a better student because she must learn to focus on her schoolwork and make better use of her time.

Many of these schools are single-sex, but coaches at those that are co-ed say that boys and girls mix easily even while being competitive with one another. Until boys' puberty kicks in with increases in testosterone, girls can more or less match them, which helps eliminate gender stereotypes, says Heather Tyrell, coach of the fifth to seventh graders at the K-8 school of Columbia University. She says, "It's not a matter of 'You got beat by a girl.' If we run 400s, the boys and girls do it together."

Callie finds the same dynamic at IS 30, where boys and girls do almost all their running as one. She says, "You never hear 'You're a girl, you can't do that.'" Gender issues have been blunted to the point where Callie will put three boys and a girl on the same relay team, and the next time around the boys will ask that the girl be included again.

With over 100 team members, intrasquad dating, and today's kids not shy about showing affection in public, Caolan Sinisi, at Marlboro, separates girls and boys by busload going to meets and sometimes has to reprimand athletes for inappropriate behavior. With a smaller group of twenty at Winston Prep, a school for grades six to twelve in the Chelsea section of Manhattan, middle school coach Allison Sheridan can keep a close eye on team relationships. "We have people dating on the team but it's not a negative," she says. "If one is going to a meet, both will go and encourage each other."

All Winston runners need encouragement because the school caters to youngsters with learning disabilities who have trouble with short-term memory and attention. "At meets," says Sheridan, who ran the New York City Marathon in 2007, "when the youngsters are divided up into their heats and lane assignments, I have to stand with them and remind them again and again to listen. They feel very insecure if they don't know what's going on."

SECURITY BLANKET SOFTENS PEER PRESSURE

In Brooklyn, coach Callie is constantly on guard for insecurity, which can surface in any facet of her team's running and behavior.

- **Performance.** At this age, many kids start out thinking that only winning is acceptable and anything else, even second, is an embarrassment and diminishes them. Disavowing this view is important for any coach or parent.

- **Discomfort.** Kids may get frightened when they sprint full-out for the first time and have to gasp for air. Growing bodies can be clumsy bodies and kids may trip and fall, suffering bruises. A hard effort might cause a youngster stomach distress and make him bring up his lunch. "I find that when I don't react in a worried manner, they calm down immediately," says Callie. However, if she gets upset, the kids do too.

- **Belonging.** More than anything, 11-to-14-year-olds desire a sense of belonging. They learn that running is special, something they can achieve that most others cannot, enhancing a sense of worth. That feeling of security is enhanced by coaches who are forthright, keeping everything aboveboard. "Kids can smell dishonesty," says Callie.

- **Options.** Most kids want to behave properly and not be led by peer pressure down the wrong path. They not only need but want boundaries. However, says Callie, "many are not aware of how to do the right thing, not aware that there are options in life. I'm giving them options. They feel safe with my options seeing their peers do it."

- **Comparisons.** Callie never compares one child with another or yells at them when they are not running as well as others. "I will never say, 'Why can't you do that the way Johnnie does?'" That will only hurt their feelings and accomplish nothing.

- **Judgments.** Callie does not talk about weight or imply that anyone is overweight. She will not point out flaws she knows the kids are sensitive to. "I find when I ignore their flaws, they feel more comfortable. They feel, 'It's okay that I'm slow.'" To that end, she does not try to correct imperfect running form, saying kids can lose interest if they don't get it right—"and why make them feel bad?"
- **Bottom line.** "The judgment we talk about centers on behavior and respect," says Callie. "It's not about your best time but the person you are. When the children finish one of our 4-mile road races they come to me looking for a hug. They want validation. They're an inspiration to me."

More evidence of the efficacy of Callie's approach comes from a parent, Jeanne Canna, when she picks up her sixth-grade boy from practice. Her older son, Justin, now a high school sophomore, ran for IS 30 for three years. His mom says, "It was absolutely great. He has identified himself as a runner and because of that stays away from smoking, drugs, alcohol. He feels no pressure because he considers himself an athlete."

If anyone wonders if Callie's style is too soft—what about those fast times a 13-year-old should aspire to?—the IS 30 trophy case is filled to capacity. Experts believe that good values make winners. "The irony," says Dr. Brenda Armstrong, of the Durham Striders youth track squad, "is if you stress healthy ideas and good values the trophies will come naturally. It's the winning attitude. Athletics is a veiled way to empower children to take control of their lives."

GIRLS CHOOSE FUN OVER PRESSURE

Research is beginning to affirm what coaches learn on the job. A 2007 study of physical activity in girls by the Tucker Center for Research on Girls and Women in Sport at the University of Minnesota found that girls enjoy activity when it's based on effort, learning, peer support, and equal treatment, and they shun activity that is "ego-oriented," favors a few, encourages competition among team members, and is generally judgmental. For girls, the study found, adult leaders and role models—parents, teachers and coaches—are critical sources of motivation and satisfaction. The study concluded that "fun is the most prevalent reason girls give for participating in sport," and that enjoyment is the strongest predictor of continued involvement.

Likewise, a six-year study of middle school girls funded by the National Heart, Lung and Blood Institute and published in the American Journal of Preventive Medicine in 2008 found that social milieu, enjoyment, and a youngster's sense of competence were "huge drivers" in making girls active in healthy forms of exercise. According to the study leader, Russ Pate, Ph.D., professor of exercise science at the University of South Carolina and perhaps the nation's foremost authority on middle school children and exercise, this was the first large-scale study to use an objective measurement of activity. "Instead of a self-report in which there's a risk that kids will tell you what you want to hear," says Pate, "we used state-of-the-art accelerometers, which are motion sensors to measure activity."

The study, the Trial of Activity in Adolescent Girls, or TAAG, was conducted in thirty-six middle schools in six states in geographically diverse areas in which more than 3,000 girls in sixth through eighth grades were assessed. Half the schools were control groups and half were given physical activity interventions. The interventions included enhancements in PE classes and establishing partnerships with community organizations that provided after-school activity to ensure continuity. "If you can change the environment in substantive ways," says Pate, a former national-caliber distance runner who competed in three Olympic trials marathons, "it will influence kids' behavior."

Activities included walking, running, and various forms of dance. Culturally tailored dance—Latin dance in a Hispanic population, for example—was most popular, according to Pate. The keys to sustained exercise for middle school girls, he says, are "make it fun and set things up so that most or all of the kids can feel successful."

Too many coaches and parents still miss the boat. They strive for little-Miss-Perfect elitism, which accounts for the high sports dropout rate—said to be as much as 70 percent—in this age-group. "When you overexpose kids to very intense training at a young age," says Pate, who has done studies of all age groups, "there's a high probability they're going to get sick of it." Pate says that personal improvement is an excellent way to frame goals and measure success. "An average kid who sets a personal best by five seconds is ecstatic," says Pate. "But ask that same youngster to win a race or even make the top ten, and he or she will feel like a failure."

Many studies focus on how to engage girls because during middle school girls, more than boys, are vulnerable to media standards that dwell on appearance and sexuality. This leads many girls to develop unhealthy attitudes with little interest in exercise. As the Tucker report states, "High social physique anxiety—feeling anxious about how others view one's body—tends to be higher in adolescent girls than in boys."

Despite the across-the-board success seen in the methods of schools like Brooklyn's IS 30, there are the polar extremes of exercise avoidance and running excess that limit girls' potential and impair health. Oftentimes, the realm of excess has an iceberg effect: you don't recognize the problem until it's too late.

EARLY STARDOM A BALANCING ACT

Some girls appear to be comfortable with fun and pressure. Jordan Hasay of Arroyo Grande, California, who made the 2008 Olympic trials 1,500-meter final as a high school junior, has been a star since seventh grade when a Web site trumpeted, "Jordan Hasay Destroys National Age 12 5K Road Best." The next year, a newspaper blared, "Hasay's Hustle: Track Phenom, 13, Among Nation's Best." Then, at 14, Hasay *was* the nation's best, winning the Foot Locker high school cross-country championship as a ninth grader, one of her many major titles against older girls and women. I've spoken with Jordan and her parents at various times. Jordan is sweet, earnest, and driven to excel. At the Olympic trials, she set a high school record of 4:14.50 and was set to enter her senior year at Mission Prep High School in the national spotlight.

Fortunately, Hasay's coach is a physician, Dr. Armando Sequeiros, a former top runner himself, who can help reduce the pressures on his protégée. For example, Sequeiros has Jordan check her resting pulse every morning. Typically, it's around 42 beats per minute. If her pulse shoots into the 50s, she does an easy day of training. "We know that patience and consistency are key. Recognize when to back off," he advises. "Listen to your body and it will tell you. Respect your body and it will guide you."

This premise guided the early running of many American women at the Beijing Games. As Beijing Olympics 10,000-meter bronze medalist Shalane Flanagan has told me: "When I was young, I looked at girls who were running faster than me and said to myself, 'I want to be that good.' But my parents held me back. They told me to be patient and always talked about long-term success. They said there was plenty of time to realize my potential."

The risks that come when young girls make the wrong choices, on or off the track, propelled a former Ironman triathlete, Molly Barker, to start the highly successful Girls on the Run program in

1996. The nonprofit enterprise for girls in grades three to eight now has 164 groups—or "councils"—throughout the United States, with some in Canada. With many sites per council (there are more than 100 sites in the northern Virginia council alone), the program has more than 40,000 girls nationwide, says Barker. She limits each group to fifteen girls to ensure personal attention from the leaders, who are more "facilitators" than coaches, in supervising a curriculum that integrates running with lessons of self-esteem, body image, and female empowerment. It's a twelve-week program done twice a year with the goal of running a 5K race. Barker divides the teaching into grades three to five and six to eight.

At the outset, Russ Pate was among the experts Barker consulted. He says, "What Molly has figured out is that you can use running as a focal point in a program with much deeper objectives. They train for a 5K, but it's really about having girls develop social skills and confidence."

With the evidence I've seen at IS 30 in Brooklyn, with the Durham Striders in North Carolina, and at Lynbrook Elementary School in Virginia that boys and girls can meld beautifully in running, I ask Pate if there's really a need for girls-only running. "Absolutely," he says. Pate points to a study he conducted with ninth-grade girls in twenty-four schools—LEAP, for Lifestyle Education of Activity Project—in which the girls who were separated by gender had greater participation in PE class than those who were mixed with boys. He says that boys and girls approach athletics differently and that in the company of boys some girls tend to feel less capable and more disengaged from the activity. Girls on the Run, he says, can better reach all girls, especially those with self-esteem issues, or what Barker calls the "girl box."

GENDER FOCUS AT GIRLS ON THE RUN

In fifth and sixth grades, says Barker, girls begin seeking attention from boys, "morphing from vibrant young women into what they think they should be," based on media and other influences. Running, she adds, takes girls out of their "boxes," providing a sanctuary. Barker, who has a master's degree in social work, says that many middle school girls are not even aware of their boxed behavior because it dominates their peer group. Running gives them healthy options, and keeping it girls-only allows for open discussion of weight, body image, and self-esteem.

Girls on the Run's holistic, nonjudgmental methods can be beneficial to any middle school youngsters seeking participation without pressure and some life lessons to go with it. The highlights:

- **Training.** The groups meet twice a week for an hour. Participants run a maximum of 3 miles. They don't keep workout logs. The girls are also encouraged to run on their own.
- **Workouts.** Runs are done as relays, games or laps of a track or field, and are structured with themes like "standing up for myself." Barker says that "social work and emotional IQ" are wrapped into the curriculum.
- **Lessons.** As an example of the above, after each completed lap girls are given an index card to hold on to and run with; afterward, while cooling off, they are asked to write "assertive statements" like "I feel angry when you call me names" for group discussion and resolution.
- **Issues.** Other themes include gossip and especially diet and eating disorders. Kids are taught to express disapproval if their moms are obsessed with weight and make comments like "I look fat in this . . ."
- **Racing.** Girls run in group-organized 5Ks or in adult events.

Some events draw large numbers of girls who are not part of Girls on the Run. The largest Girls on the Run 5K, in northern Virginia, has over 2,000 participants. While about a third of Girls on the Run youngsters are competitive, says Barker, there's a fun run approach, with every participant receiving a racing bib emblazoned with the number 1.

- **Bottom line.** Running is used to celebrate a girl's strengths while overcoming "shame-based" attitudes in which middle school girls feel, "There's something wrong with me."

With running required only forty-eight days a year, can girls be influenced in the profound ways that Girls on the Run seeks, especially in the upper age group, which is confronted by so many diversions? Barker says that 40 to 50 percent of the girls return from year to year and testing in the form of questionnaires, given before and after the programs, shows that girls' self-esteem, body image, and intrinsic motivation to be active all increase.

From a training standpoint, twenty-four weeks a year is quite sufficient, says Pate, to learn about running and experience improvement in fitness. He maintains that for most kids this age, "year-round training is too much in every way you would interpret it." He says kids should get "wide exposure" to activity, from basketball and soccer to swimming and rock climbing.

Barker says she will soon launch a longitudinal study that follows their girls after eighth grade and into high school and adulthood. In the meantime, her new program, Sole Mates, will engage high school runners to serve as mentors to the younger Girls on the Run participants.

Great idea. High school runners from the front lines know that most kids do well with a light touch. At Marlboro, coach Sinisi plays to kids' funny bones with "long and lovely" workouts, easy runs of three to four miles. Kids come up to her asking, "Can we run long and lovely today?"

WHO ATE MY RUNNING SHOES?

Cherish that eagerness. When you're working with middle school runners, says Sinisi, be prepared for a "crazy time in the life of a child."

- **Learning curve.** "I tell parents that their child has to learn how to learn, in class and in running. They lack the ability because of peer pressure." She says kids' focus is compromised by the influence of friends who, for example, may regard certain stretching exercises as "dorky."
- **"The cat ate my running shoes."** Be prepared for team members to forget not only their running shoes but running shorts, water bottle—everything they need. Instead of berating them, go lightly, says Sinisi, letting them learn from mistakes.
- **Go lightly, but not too lightly.** Sinisi criticizes parents who let their kids quit the team without a fight, and those who readily provide excuses for their kids when they miss practice for no good reason.
- **When excuses are okay.** Running should not be full-time and youngsters should try everything. "I am okay with a kid missing practice to go to chorus or band," says Sinisi, "just as their music teachers have to be okay with the student missing a class for a meet."
- **Big shots.** She says a coach should never say to a middle school girl on a track squad, "I bet you'd be a great shot putter." That is the ultimate embarrassment, which, Sinisi says, the girl will take as, *You're a big girl and I want you to throw heavy things around for me*. (The answer to that dilemma may be to ask a small but strong—or at least willing—girl. At IS 30, coach Callie has a couple of sixth-grade girls doing the shot put. They also run the 100 meters. Sprinting is their gig, but they're team players and the shot could mean

extra points. And throwing an iron ball around can be fun. Context matters.)

In Brooklyn, at Leif Erickson Park, what matters during IS 30's sprint work is (1) cutting from an outside lane to the inside to shave distance and get competitive position, (2) learning to push hard and not give up, like Estrella says, and (3) relaxing and taking deep breaths between runs.

As the kids run, Callie calls out, "If you see a hole to the inside, take it." She says some meets do not have staggered starts and kids positioned on the outside are at a disadvantage. The fastest boys run their 200s in 32 seconds; the top girls do 36. One Muslim girl wears a hijab. "Breathe," says Callie. "In through the nose, out the mouth." She tells me that when the kids get excited they clench their teeth and hold their breath. "They need to be reminded to breathe."

If a 13-year-old forgets fundamentals, he or she can still be counted on to appreciate the bigger picture. When Callie takes the team indoors in the dead of winter and shows a film about the late Oregon running star Steve Prefontaine (nicknamed Pre), the kids' favorite part, she says, is when Pre wins a race, then takes off his shoes to reveal feet bloodied by blisters.

Whether inspired by their coach, whose first name refers to the ancient Greeks' Muse of epic poetry, or by the legend of Pre, the IS 30 runners do their park sprints like there's no tomorrow. Their practice is seamless. Their cool-down walk back to school is a joy. The runners talk amiably and on the last block, on an uphill stretch, they break into a run and race back to where it all began.

▶ **Should Middle School Runners Compete on High School Teams? A National Debate**

At least a dozen states allow seventh and eighth graders to join high school track and cross-country programs under certain circumstances. Oftentimes, these athletes, especially on the girls' side, make the varsity squad and even star on the team. New York is prominent among the states in seeing middle school girls lead high school teams to statewide and national standing.

In New York, the rule, called "selective classification," is a regulation of the State Education Department and applies to all sports. "The philosophy behind it," says Bob Stulmaker, assistant director of the New York State Public High Schools Athletic Association, "is for seventh and eighth graders who display physical skills and body maturation to compete at a higher level."

Students must get medical clearance from a school doctor who evaluates physical maturity. They also must pass a skills test composed of a standing long jump, shuttle run, flex arm hang, curl-ups, and 1.5-mile timed run. "It's athletics' version of AP classes or 'enrichment,'" says Matt Jones of the Shenendehowa school district, north of Albany. Jones was Shenendehowa High's track and cross-country coach for twenty years, and also the school's athletic director for ten years. His teams won many state and national honors.

Jones believes that selective classification is good for advanced youngsters as long as it's handled properly. As a coach, he designated an assistant to supervise the middle school runners with a toned-down training program and low-key racing. Jones points out that many middle schools don't have a regular track program, and kids who want to run may have no option other than a high school team.

How can youngsters' well-being be safeguarded? Can they be brought along properly, even if some coaches want to rush their progress for team points and some parents are happy to see their "future stars" in the spotlight? "When I talk to seventh- through ninth-grade coaches," says Jones, "I tell them the number one priority is that the kids have fun and return the following year. It's not always about personal bests but developing basic skills and exposing them to techniques like baton passing. Make sure they finish the season with a smile on their faces."

One issue that Jones and others cite is that of the immature girl of 12 or 13 being in the midst of socially savvy 17- and 18-year-old girls. Even riding together on a bus to a meet can be treacherous for the youngster. The same is true for boys. Stulmaker alerts parents to this matter. Aggressive coaching also concerns him. "If the program is run properly, for the gifted, physically mature athlete, then it's a good program. If it's used to fill rosters, then that's an abuse of the program."

Stulmaker was formerly athletic director at Saratoga Springs High School, which has made substantial use of middle school runners in its girls' cross-country team, ranked number one or two in the nation twelve of the last sixteen years. A recent example is Nicole Blood, who began setting records in seventh grade. To some, her aggressive pace seemed risky, but now, at the University of Oregon, she is one of the nation's top collegians and an academic all-American to boot.

"I would hold Nicole up as the ideal," says Jennifer Fazioli, 27, an assistant coach at Albany State who traveled the same path in seventh grade at Averill Park High. Fazioli had been running with her father and said the middle school program was inadequate. She ran well in high school and said that when she was 12 the older girls embraced her. "We used to joke that the 18-year-olds could have been my babysitters."

It's not only the age factor but developmental differences that concern Russ Pate, Ph.D., the University of South Carolina middle school expert. "Some kids are prepubescent, some pubescent, some even postpubescent," he says. "Puberty is not always kind to girls. They should not be overexposed to a highly competitive environment too early."

Other high school coaches from around the country weigh in:

Art Keene, Amherst Regional High School, Amherst, Massachusetts

"Massachusetts allows seventh and eighth graders if they are in the same building with the high school population, or under the administration of the same principal. The idea has merits. We run against small schools that would be unable to fill a squad if not for the younger kids. These athletes get attached to running before being distracted by less wholesome activities. They are mentored by older runners. Coaching should be sensible and the young kids not brought along too quickly."

Adam Kedge, Albuquerque Academy, Albuquerque, New Mexico

"New Mexico allows eighth graders to compete on a high school program on a district basis. Kids who get involved early can start to develop good conditioning. Where there are no middle school sports, kids get an opportunity. However, overzealous adults can ruin any good idea, and eighth graders should not be pushed beyond what is right for their age. A good example for us was an 800 runner who ran 1:56 in eighth grade. Keeping him in middle school competition would have been unfair to him and his peers."

Jim Kilbreth, Spartanburg High School, Spartanburg, South Carolina

"South Carolina allows seventh and eighth graders to run in high school in noncontact sports. It has been good for cross-country, preparing the youngsters for the hard work beginning in ninth grade. The kids get hooked on running early and start excelling as freshmen if they are brought along properly. Dealing with lack of maturity is important. Some youngsters have difficulty practicing every day. Coaches must be patient."

Chad Waggoner, Trinity High School, Louisville, Kentucky

"If the middle school is a feeder school to the high school, Kentucky allows the younger athletes to take part. Usually you see this in smaller rural schools; some kids are as young as sixth grade. I don't like the idea. While the youngsters may help fill a roster, many of them seem to burn out by the end of high school. This is used mostly with girls who start off great when they're lightweight but are no longer out front when they start to develop physically."

Dave Zittleman, Bismarck High School, Bismarck, North Dakota

"The policy is allowed statewide, and you see more girls moving up than boys. I like the idea and feel the youngsters should run some middle school meets along with varsity events. Some of our smaller schools would not be able to field a team without seventh and eighth graders. However, the success of some of the young girls, in particular, does not always come as easily in the upper grades, and they feel frustrated training just as hard but not seeing the same results as their bodies mature."

David Bloor, St. Catherine's High School, Richmond, Virginia

"Girls start coming out for our high school team as sixth graders. They run three or four days a week, 10 to 20 miles total. My older girls do 30 to 35 a week. I have had dozens of girls run all seven years, grades six through twelve, with a wide range of ability, but all with enthusiasm. One 1995 graduate returned to address the student body. She said that while she never won a race or even placed, she learned a great deal about perseverance and dedication and had just finished her first marathon."

On the Run: A Primer for Ages 12 to 14

Starting out. Middle schools typically have a cross-country season in the fall and track season in spring. It's good to do some summer running to prepare for fall. Youngsters need to learn proper pacing and become comfortable with pushing hard in practice and meets. Experiment with different distances to see which ones you prefer.

Healthy fun. Do a variety of sports as opposed to specializing in running year-round. Youngsters should feel fresh and eager and motivated. If practices are held daily, that's plenty of running. If there are only a couple of practices per week, fill in with running on days off.

Must-do stretches. With big growth spurts, kids this age need to maintain flexibility. To stretch the groin area, sit on the ground with legs spread and knees straight and lean forward bringing head toward the ground. For the hamstring muscles in the back of the legs, stand with right foot over left and, keeping knees straight, try to touch toes.

Fail-safe workouts. Cross-country training should always include some hill running on grassy fields, found at school facilities and parks. Youngsters should run for a half hour or more while pushing up hills. In track, run 4 to 8 × 300 meters at a brisk pace; after each 300, jog 100 back to start, then walk a little for about 3 minutes' rest between runs.

Helpful parents. Parental support is best shown at competitions. Cheer for your youngsters but not overly so, which could prove embarrassing. At this age, peer acceptance informs everything, so give your young teen plenty of space and save any "silly" questions for back home.

Running distances. Cross-country races are typically 1.5 miles, more or less. They could be 3K, or 3,000 meters (1.8 miles). Track covers all distances from the 100-meter sprint up through

3,200 meters (about 2 miles), plus the hurdles and field events. In the off-season an occasional road race can help keep kids involved. Here are some suggested distance/time ranges:

Age	Distance and Frequency
12	3 miles or 30 minutes three to five days a week
13	4 miles or 40 minutes three to five days a week
14	5 miles or 50 minutes three to five days a week

Miles Per Week: New team members can gain a lot of fitness on as little as 10 miles a week. Eighth graders, especially those who plan to run in high school, can work up to about 20 miles a week, but only for certain periods, not year-round. Boys and girls are the same.

Racing by age. This age group also enjoys racing. Suggested race distances:

Age	Race Distance
12	Sprints to 5K (3.1 miles)
13	Sprints to 5K (3.1 miles)
14	Sprints to 5K (3.1 miles) or 10K (6.2 miles)

Target mile times. These provide safe, comfortable goals.

Age	Boys' Target	Girls' Target
12	6:30–7:00	7:00–7:30
13	6:00–6:30	6:30–7:00
14	5:30–6:00	6:00–6:30

7

Running with the Female Body

The athlete should feel confident that she deserves to get what she wants out of running. The reason she is running is that it brings joy, health, freedom to her.

—Arianna Lambie, former national high school champion
from Massachusetts and Stanford All-American

In the fall of 1993, I learned of a long-term study of injury patterns among 60,000 high school athletes in eighteen sports in the Seattle area. It was conducted from 1979 to 1992 and was the most comprehensive research of its kind to that point. The study covered sports by gender, so there were different sets of statistics—for example, in boys' soccer versus girls' soccer. Indeed, no research as encompassing on high school sports injuries has been done since.

Like anyone who followed athletics, I would have expected then that contact sports such as football and basketball, or perhaps a sport such as gymnastics in which youngsters leapt through the air with crash landings, would have shown the highest incidence of injury. But when I interviewed Dr. Stephen G. Rice, the physician who conducted the study, I was startled to learn that girls' cross-country running was a clear-cut number one, ahead of football and wrestling. Dr. Rice, then director of the Athletic Health Care System at the University of Washington and a specialist in pediatric and orthopedic sports medicine, found that girls' cross-country had 61.4 injuries per 100 athletes. Football, at number two, had 58.8, while wrestling, number three, had 49.7. Girls' soccer, number four, had 43.7, and boys' cross-country, number five, had 38.7.

With boys' cross-country injury rates about 63 percent of what girls showed, the factors behind the alarming girls' injury rate were clearly not about cross-country itself but emphatically about gender. As further evidence of female distance runners' apparent vulnerability to injury, girls' track and field was number nine at 24.8 injuries per 100 athletes and boys' track was number thirteen at 17.3. Track and field has sprints, hurdles, and field events requiring explosive movements that are associated with high injury risk. Girls' cross-country, considered easygoing compared to running the 100 meters or high jumping, had more than twice the injury rate of girls' track and more than three times the injury rate of boys' track.

Dr. Rice told me then that even though the findings were limited to the Seattle area, he felt that they were indicative of a national trend. While the results surprised me, they led me to think of the many individual cases of injured young female distance runners I'd come across—all of them extremely thin—as I covered the sport. Many of these girls were trumpeted as future stars and inevitably hailed as "the next Mary Decker" after the precocious 1970s teen who went on to set numerous records and become a world champion.

GIRLS' HEALTH ISSUES BECOME A NATIONAL TREND

When I proceeded to write a *New York Times* story on the Seattle study and its implications, I found that Dr. Rice's view of the national picture was on target: doctors, exercise physiologists, and coaches all said that increasing numbers of girls around the country were getting injured from intense running programs at a young age and that they were pressured by parents to earn college scholarships and by aggressive coaches ill-informed about the complex nature of girls' adolescent development.

As related to running, girls' developmental issues involved caloric intake, nutrition, body weight, anatomy, hormonal changes, menstruation, energy expenditure, body image, family dynamics, and the way our society and the athletic community regard children and females in particular—indeed, the whole of a young girl's existence. These issues were not easily understood—especially by parents blinded by their youngsters' initial success, well-meaning coaches gung-ho on motivating promising talent, and media looking for a good story on the next superstar.

What is most important to emphasize is that distance running is absolutely wonderful for young girls in every respect—no less so than it is for boys—but that girls' particular development and maturation are best nurtured by a low-key training and racing approach in the younger age group. This is especially important for girls who show early success. They can easily be captured by the whirlwind of the track and cross-country circuit and thrust into an accelerated program with short-term gains but long-term peril.

There are no risks in erring on the side of caution, in giving a girl less running at first; she can always make it up later on, make huge progress, and fulfill her potential. But there is risk in doing too much too soon. The risks impact not only running but overall health.

A young girl's early running "talent" can be misleading. There is not a single example of a child star becoming a professional star. (Mary Decker doesn't count. She was a teen before Title IX—before a plethora of national youth and high school events, high-priced athletic scholarships for women, and over-the-top sports parenting.) At the same time, if you look at today's American female professionals, you'll find that the top performers all took a restrained, long-term approach in their youth.

My *Times* story, "Girls' Cross-Country Takes Heavy Toll, Study Shows," ran on the newspaper's front page on December 4, 1993. Other page-one subjects that day included the national unemployment rate, Iran-contra, space shuttle dangers, and a double teenage suicide on Long Island. The *Times* felt that the "wow" factor of girls' running injuries surpassing those of football, along with how accelerated training of young girls affected their healthy development, was the kind of national trend worthy of attention. Girls' sports in general were growing in participation and recognition while acquiring some of the same abuses affecting high-profile boys' sports, and the *Times* and other media tried to keep pace.

Seeing more and more girls victimized by running too much too soon, I continued scrutinizing female running trends while alerting people in the sport to the hazards facing overzealous, fleet-footed girls. The girls themselves were not responsible for their difficulties, and certainly not for their ambition, which was commendable. It was the adults in charge who needed to take a step back.

INCREASED INTENSITY IMPERILS RUNNERS

From what I've observed, little has changed in the decade and a half since the Seattle report. When I revisited the subject with Dr. Rice in 2006, he told me, "I think the data still stand. It's a reflection of the way in which young athletes are trained. Today, people are even more intense than they were back then." Rice is currently director of the Jersey Shore Sports Medicine Center at University Medical Center in Neptune, in Monmouth County, where I live. "Today," he said, "we have year-round sports, a lot of overuse. It's the nature of society. We're trying to make kids grow up faster. We're almost 'stealing' their childhood with so much structured time."

In our ramped-up, resume-building culture in which kids are programmed without a minute to spare, the "end of childhood" is hardly news. But maybe it's gotten worse than we'd realized. In many overachieving families, there seem to be two parallel ideas in raising girls: having it all and being perfect. Young girls should not have to be burdened by such expectations.

In running, the young female is looked at differently than her male counterparts. Boys can screw up and still be loved. In fact, boys can be loved *for* screwing up. Let their silly machismo, considered a passing stage, run its course. I get the sense that girls feel a need to earn their stripes by reaching for the stars at every turn. Their families depend on it. The female runner is their prize. But as an embodiment of strength and beauty, of athletic power and lithe speed, the female runner is also *our* prize.

Maybe that's why a leading New Jersey high school girls track and cross-country coach, Brian Zatorski of Southern Regional in Manahawkin, told me one day when I watched his practice session that in his view girls who run will "suffer" more readily than boys. Girls, he said, will always run to the limit, even asking for more work, while boys will look for shortcuts. In this scenario, girls are more "macho" than boys. Zatorski has seen this tendency in girls with average talent as well as with two national girls' champions he's coached in the mile run. Why? The need to please, he suggests.

The girl as success symbol has also impressed Peter Martin, who coaches girls' cross-country at Newton North High outside Boston, one of the top academic high schools in the country. The school was featured in a front-page *New York Times* story in 2007, titled, "For Girls, It's Be Yourself, and Be Perfect, Too." In a 5,000-word piece, North's über-girls were put under the microscope, and I felt both admiration and sadness for many of them. One 17-year-old was described as "a great student, classical pianist, fluent in Spanish, and a three-season varsity runner and track captain." Martin told the *Times'* writer, Sara Rimer, "that girls try so hard to please everyone—coaches, teachers, parents— that he bends over backward not to criticize them." He said, "I tell them, 'Just go out and run.'"

Other girls' teams could probably do well with that approach. Distance running for large numbers of girls is relatively new, dating back to the 1970s when Title IX was legislated. From the standpoint of what constitutes healthy approaches for competition, girls' running is still undergoing experimentation and growing pains.

GIRLS' ELITE PRODUCES MIXED RESULTS

Many accepted measures of excellence are ambiguous. The Foot Locker high school national cross-country championship, established in 1979, is considered a stepping-stone for the elite teen athletes who qualify for the event. For boys, it has been. But for girls' winners the future has been mixed; no titlist, for example, has ever gone on to capture the NCAA cross-country title.

I have been personally inspired by mature, healthy-looking young girls running with coltish grace and power. I have also been frightened by ultrathin, twiglike females running a cross-country course. These latter girls are sitting ducks for stress fractures, which doctors say are epidemic among aggressive female runners.

Adult leadership must be held accountable. Every female runner has a right to progress at her own rate, have health and reproductive issues taken into account, and be nurtured for long-term fitness and well-being. Running yourself ragged can result from too many training miles, too fast a pace too often, too many races, too much pressure to perform, too little rest, inadequate food intake, and more.

A recent college graduate, Arianna Lambie, originally from Massachusetts, is a potential Olympian who embodies the correct approach. On a modest program, Lambie was the national high school mile champion in 2003. After that, she was a fourteen-time all-American at Stanford. In 2007, Lambie told me, "I was lucky enough to have parents and coaches who saw the long-term goals." Asked for her view of what the young female runner needs most, Lambie replied, "The athlete should feel confident that she deserves to get what *she* wants out of running. The reason she is running is that it brings joy, health, freedom to *her*."

I believe this freedom is compromised in many instances by the dichotomy of the child-woman—the blurred sexuality of the young female runner evolving into womanhood, secure at first in the perfect form of her childness in flight and then confronting new contradictions and conflicts over her maturing body. I watch these kids run like the wind and see a kind of purity, an ideal, something that exalts human promise. It feels precious. But nature has a say.

There is the overtrained girl who develops Swiss cheese bones from a combination of low body fat, caloric deficit, delayed menstruation, and lack of desperately needed estrogen, and consequently is forced to the sidelines with one injury after another. And there is the girl on the fast track who develops her pubescent curves, adds body fat and weight, and slows down, her self-image shattered by being surpassed by the young twigs next in line.

GIRLS' DEVELOPMENT AND RUNNING

Here are important factors at the intersection of girls' development and running, with measures to ease the process.

BODY TALK

Female runners' development issues tend to be avoided because they may be considered private matters. "It's always the elephant in the room in our sport," said Ed Purpura, girls' cross-country coach at 2005 Maryland state champion Severna Park, in a 2006 *Washington Post* article by Eli Saslow on physiological factors that slow girls down. "Nobody likes to talk about it." In the same story, a club coach, Brian Funk, was said to take the initiative, "asking every girl he coaches about her menstrual cycle." Saslow wrote, "Sometimes the conversations feel awkward but they allow him to gauge an athlete's sustenance."

Another coach with the right idea is John Barr of Texas, former girls' track and cross-country coach of state winner Kingwood High. "Make sure you know girls' relevant health history prior to high school," he advises.

Girls in the United States, on average, get their periods at age 11 or 12. For runners the average is closer to fourteen, according to doctors. If a female runner has not reached puberty by thirteen, she should be checked out by her physician, says Dr. Mona Shangold, director of the Center for Women's Health and Sports Gynecology in Philadelphia. Aside from the age touchstone, Dr. Shangold said it's advisable for girls in running "to check growth with their pediatrician on a regular basis. There's a fine line between normal and excessive stress in running."

Bottom line: Girls should have a comfort level discussing their adolescent development.

BUILDING BONE

The years following puberty are a time of rapid bone formation for adolescent females. Girls build 60 to 80 percent of their skeletal mass by 18. For bone to build, it must be nourished with sufficient nutrients. Female runners who do not take in enough calories may have an "athletic energy deficit," which commonly results in stress fractures and can cause long-term health issues, according to experts. A caloric deficit can also delay the onset of menstruation, setting off a chain reaction of recurrent health and running problems.

Girls with suspected bone issues should take a bone density test, according to Dr. Angela Smith, an orthopedist at Children's Hospital of Philadelphia who has treated many young athletes. The test is an X-ray and the cost is about $300. Dr. Smith recommends taking the test at a children's hospital, as opposed to a local lab, to ensure expert analysis. "The best way to achieve healthy bone density," she said, "is to eat a healthy diet, taking in sufficient calories and including key nutrients like calcium and zinc."

A growing preteen should take in 20 calories per pound of body weight, plus the calories burned in daily activity, according to Dr. Bill Roberts, former president of the American College of Sports Medicine. For a 100-pound girl running five miles a day, that's at least 2,500 calories.

Bottom line: Girls should take in sufficient calories to ensure healthy bone growth.

HELPING HORMONES

In a caloric deficit, girls will not start a new function like reproduction, said Dr. Smith, and this leads to deficient production of the hormone estrogen. "Lack of estrogen," says Dr. Shangold, "prevents the formation of additional bone and accelerates the loss of bone." Girls who go through their formative years with insufficient bone are predisposed to develop adult osteoporosis as early as their 30s.

Excess thinness, low body fat, poor eating, and overdoing it in running combine to put the young runner at high risk of poor bone health. "Too little energy and too much repetitive pounding," says Smith. She gave an example of a female patient who was on the high school track team and training with the varsity. The girl had not yet developed her reproductive functioning and was at an age of rapid growth. She was very fast, so the coach gave her extra workouts. "She ended up with stress fractures in her legs and could not finish the season," said Dr. Smith.

Bottom line: Girls should know that poor health habits can result in running injuries.

GROWING PAINS

The early teens are also a time of a girl's "peak height velocity." During this phase, said Dr. Smith, the girl is growing most rapidly and can be hurt by sudden increases in training. "Bones are growing long—the early bone, the pre-bone—but that bone has not yet solidly mineralized and remodeled into the good, strong structure the girl is going to eventually have," explained Dr. Smith. In addition, because the growth is rapid, flexibility and strength of the muscles does not keep pace and, said Dr. Smith, "the girl is at a period of maximum risk in terms of muscle, bone, tendon, and ligament growth—and at the same time a major change in training load is often imposed."

At this age as well, girls become gangly, uncoordinated, and "lose their sense of space," said Dr. Smith. Girls temporarily lose running efficiency and don't run "evenly," putting undue stress on the knees and ankles. This awkwardness results from a widening of girls' hips while the long femur bones in the upper leg pull farther apart, creating an angle, explained Dr. Oded Bar-Or, professor of pediatrics and director of the Children's Exercise and Nutrition Center at McMaster University in Ontario, Canada.

Bottom line: Girls should know that normal growth can result in awkward running posture.

GENDER GAP

Puberty makes boys better athletes because rising testosterone levels make boys bigger and stronger. In contrast, puberty oftentimes makes girls "worse" athletes, temporarily, because rising estrogen concentrations make girls bigger and heavier. On average, a girl going through puberty gains 10 to 20 pounds. Excess fat is a hindrance in running as in many other sports.

Until puberty, girls have 90 percent of the aerobic capacity that boys have, said Dr. Smith. This is a key reason why ultrathin preteen girls excel in distance running. But, as we've seen, it's an artificial advantage. The pursuit of high performance at this age must be weighed against the risk of diminished performance with weight gain.

Bottom line: Girls should accept weight gain and body fat as part of normal development.

MENSTRUATION

Health professionals say that a girl requires at least 17 percent body fat in order to menstruate, the key signal of a girl's natural, healthy growth. "The menstrual period is like the canary in the coal mine," says Dr. Smith. "It's a sign that all systems are working and a girl has enough energy." An irregular menstrual cycle is often combined with disordered eating and weak bones—the "female athletic triad"—to create havoc. "Every day in my office, I see at least one girl who fits the definition of menstrual disturbance," said Dr. Smith, who defined that condition as six or fewer periods a year. "That's when I start getting really worried."

Dr. Smith said that girls should have their first period no later than two years after the start of breast development. Girls who are late should be examined by a gynecologist. Menstrual bleeding, says Dr. Shangold, is an indication that a girl is making estrogen and progesterone, necessary for bone building and good health in general. She also says that it's okay for girls to run and race during menstruation. "Girls can take over-the-counter medication to alleviate menstrual cramps and reduce bleeding. Using tampons is also desirable," she says.

Bottom line: Girls should be aware of menstruation's role in running performance.

STRESS FRACTURES

When natural development is stalled, injuries such as stress fractures are almost inevitable. At minimum, stress fractures in the lower leg, for example, require a six-week layoff, which could end a season. It is not uncommon for girls who have one stress fracture to experience repeated injuries. Bones are most likely to break during rapid growth periods, said Dr. Smith. Oftentimes, the fractures occur toward the end of the bones, the point of fastest growth.

One highly public example of repeated injury occurred with Julia Stamps of California, one of the most heralded young runners of the past twenty years. After winning the Foot Locker cross-country title as a high school sophomore in 1994, she did not finish the national event in 1995 and '96. Still, Stamps went on to Stanford on a track scholarship. But she was repeatedly sick and injured, the result, she told me, of amenorrhea, or lack of menstruation, stemming from intense training.

Stamps' nadir came in the fall of her senior year at Stanford. In pain, she did not race all season but still competed in the NCAA cross-country meet to help her team. The wind-chill was −15° in Ames, Iowa. "Afterward," Stamps told me, "I could hardly walk. The diagnosis was a stress fracture in the sacrum."

Dr. Smith said that girls who have had repeated stress fractures and decide to eat more may still not get their periods for a while but *will* begin to heal better. "We see a quantum improvement in healing when they finally get their period," she said. "Whether that's related to eating or the additional impetus of estrogen, nobody knows."

Bottom line: Girls should be aware of the consequences of caloric deficit.

HEALTHY BUT SLOWER

Menstruation is a double-edged sword. While girls' bodies change in healthy ways, their bodies also change in a manner incongruent with fast running in the short term. As stated, girls gain weight and fat. They also put on some muscle. In some girls, there is a decrease in iron stores. "Hemoglobin level in the blood goes down during puberty in girls," says Dr. Bar-Or. With this drop, the capacity of the blood to carry oxygen is reduced, a significant performance deterrent.

Bottom line: Girls should learn to accept performance fluctuations associated with development.

IRON LOSS

Loss of iron through menstrual bleeding, poor diet, and heavy running can cause an iron deficiency, impairing performance. "Low iron affects oxygen delivery and you'll tire and be out of breath," says Dr. Todd Fowler, a Johnson City, Tennessee, sports medicine specialist. "You can also get aching, numbness, and muscle cramping. When you drink, you dilute the blood even more, because you restock fluids but don't restock iron. Then you feel worse."

High mileage is another factor. "Every time your foot strikes the ground," says Fowler, "you 'kill' little blood vessels in the bottom of your foot."

A few years ago, a college freshman who'd starred in high school found that with increased training she suffered from fatigue, headaches, and dizziness. A blood test showed that she had a low level of ferritin, a protein that binds to iron to store it in the liver. On doctor's orders, she took iron supplements and began eating iron-rich foods like red meat. She resumed easy running and within a few months was back to normal.

Girls with similar symptoms should consider getting blood work. Take both a CBC test for hemoglobin and a serum ferritin test because hemoglobin can be normal while ferritin can still be low.

Bottom line: Girls should have iron levels checked if they experience undue fatigue.

EMOTIONAL LOWS

For girls, a drop in performance after exceptional early success, whether related to delaying womanhood or reaching it, can be devastating. Alison Smith, a three-time state cross-country winner in Maryland, faced the latter. "You get heavier and hit a plateau where you stop improving," she told the *Washington Post*. "You lose focus and it's like, 'How can I ever fix this?'"

The frustration is toughest on the marquee runners because they shoulder the most pressure and team responsibility and confront a deeper performance drop. And there's always the college scholarship at stake. Until the slowdown, a girl may well have been considered "perfect" by all concerned, even by herself.

In an interview, one high school all-American told me that as a sophomore she had "anorexic tendencies," referring to the eating disorder anorexia nervosa. She was rail-thin at 5 foot 8 and 100 pounds. She trained up to 50 miles a week and said she took in a mere 500 calories a day. Then, before her junior year, she experienced the growth spurt that Dr. Smith talked about, shooting up to 5 foot 10. As a result, her performances suffered and her spirit flagged. After finally improving her diet to take in adequate calories, she accepted her growing body and slower race times because she felt healthier and knew that her running would improve in due time.

Bottom line: Girls should avoid comparisons with other runners and focus on healthy growth.

EMOTIONAL HIGHS

Coaches say that girls are motivated to run their best when performance goals are balanced with making friends on the team and creating a network of support so the training and racing are only part of the running experience. Girls tend to thrive when the atmosphere is purposeful but relaxed and there is no favoritism given to elite runners. Girls also enjoy running most when camaraderie is emphasized with team socials, and when an athlete's commitment is stressed for the benefit of the team on the whole. Girls respond to a family setting much more than when individual glory is stressed.

One team that embodies this approach is Los Alamos High in the Jemez mountains of northern New Mexico. When I visited the Hilltoppers a few years ago for insights into their many state and national honors, I spoke with some of the varsity girls cross-country runners, who had this to say about what they enjoyed most: "Running with friends." (Brittany Somers) "Everybody knows your 'pain' so you have a bond with other people that most other sports don't have." (Kate Preteska) "You become close, like a family." (Anna Miller) "Running makes you happy. You are with people who are cheery, not grumpy." (Analisa Sandoval).

▶ The Joy of Running in Good Health

Here's how to make sure all girls experience the joys of running as they grow through the teen years.

1. **Communication.** Maintain open and honest communication so that girls feel comfortable expressing their feelings, positive or negative, about their running with parents, siblings, coaches, teammates, and health professionals. Girls may say they enjoy hard training to please adults or out of fear of being judged negatively.

2. **Training.** Running a few miles a day a few days a week facilitates enjoyment and good health without undue pressure in the years before high school.

3. **Eating.** Healthy eating should be nurtured along with healthy running so that girls develop a complete picture of what's involved in feeling good and having a sense of well-being.

4. **Medical.** Make regular doctor visits to check on growth and puberty issues while enlisting the pediatrician as part of the family team.

5. **Body image.** Do not promote thinness as an ideal or dis-

cuss stereotypical cover-girl beauty as a goal. Healthy running and eating and the glow of contentment will make every girl "beautiful."

6. Team emphasis. Emphasize team over individual goals and include social activities like pasta parties and other bonding experiences.

7. Stereotypes. For some girls, bonding with other girls in a values-based instructional environment such as Girls on the Run helps mitigate harmful stereotypes. (See chapter 6 for more about Girls on the Run.)

8. Sisterhood. In a nonjudgmental, girls-only environment, some females may feel more liberated to take on hard challenges. Dr. Jennifer Sluder, a pediatrician at Childrens Hospital Los Angeles, told me that when 700 teenage girls in the Students Run LA marathon program were given additional girls-only goals of running a 5K or 10K, they were less likely to drop out of the marathon program.

9. Long-term approach. Do not promote the idea that heavy training and child stardom will lead to unimpeded glory for years to come. A girl on a high school team should do her best running in her senior year and have plenty of life in her legs—and desire in her heart—for running in college, if she chooses, or on her own.

10. Adolescent changes. Emphasize that all adolescents go through changes—that testosterone gives boys muscle mass while estrogen gives girls body fat. "The context of *everyone* changing makes it more palatable to girls," says Dr. Susan Carter, a gynecological surgeon on the medical staff at the 2008 Olympic track and field trials who also coaches girls' cross-country at Greeley West High School in Colorado.

11. The big picture. Be careful about emphasizing a championship event, says Dr. Carter, because "it's too much pressure to be 'on' for one event at a point in time." Your performance "should not define you as an athlete or person. Always look at the big picture."

12. Competition. Top-performing girls may compete in three or even four events in state meets, running the 800, 1,600, 3,200, and perhaps 4 × 800 relay. "This is an awful practice," according to Dr. Michael E. Sargent, a sports medicine specialist in the Department of Orthopedics of Vermont School of Medicine. "At one meet, a girl had been told that she'd 'only' have to double but the coach put her in a third event without her knowledge. She burst into tears, shouting, 'I hate track.' She did not mean the endeavor of running" but participating in a program so insensitive to her needs.

13. Specialization. Young girls should do a variety of sports and avoid "full-time" running until at least sophomore or junior year of high school. Year-round sports specialization is at the crux of the proliferation of girls' injuries and health issues, says Dr. Angela Smith, and why an estimated 70 percent of girls quit sports by their teen years.

Julia Stamps almost suffered that same fate. Referring to her high school experience she said, "It became, 'Can you beat yourself?' I tried to compete against myself, but you can't do that day in and day out. You need a break. I had a lot of other interests that I wanted to pursue but was not able to."

But even Stamps' ordeal has had a happy ending. Today, after years of injury and frustration, she is a successful marathon runner in her late twenties, married and having a child, with a career in the finance field. Once told she would never run again, unable to walk, and sidelined for over a year, she now runs free of pain.

8

Running with the Male Ego

Boys measure everything they do or say by a single yardstick: does this make me look weak? And if it does, they're not going to do it.

—MICHAEL THOMPSON, AUTHOR OF *Raising Cain*

The first thing I noticed when I started coaching a boys' cross-country team at a New Jersey high school in the late 1990s was the girls' squad. At practice, these young ladies listened attentively to the coach's instructions, spoke politely with one another, and seemed to enjoy each phase of the training session. They wore regulation running clothes, had their requisite water bottles lined up in readiness, and sat in a perfect circle as they stretched their leg muscles for the run along the boardwalk on the Jersey Shore. I took their attitude as a sign of the maturity expected of student-athletes. These teenage girls understood that in their efforts they would fulfill a responsibility not only to themselves but to team, school, coach, family—and perhaps even God, since this was a Catholic school.

Oh, the shock when my boys arrived at our practice site and behaved like prison inmates on a break in the exercise yard. They scowled and shoved one another, staked out their turf, ignored me, disobeyed me, cursed, and got into mischief when they thought I wasn't looking. Not one youngster gave the impression that he wanted to be a member of the St. Rose High School Purple Roses cross-country team.

As I gazed in frustration at the ocean waves while my boys stumbled out to their training runs, I thought: *What's wrong with boys?* Why was it more important for the seniors on the squad, who I'd assumed would be leaders and role models, to toss a nerdy freshman into the water instead of rallying the younger boys to work harder on a 5-mile run?

I should have known the answer. After all, I was a boy once. As a teenager in the early 1960s I also ran on a high school cross-country team. If the coach took his eye off us, we played football. Our priority was fooling around, not running around.

Those images stuck with me. Things only got worse that first fall season. While the straight-arrow girls' team trained hard and marched to victory, I had to threaten boys with expulsion for misbehavior or for being found in the school gym playing basketball when they were supposed to be running. It was the same lack of control I experienced as a young New York City middle school teacher in 1969 when I took over in midsemester for a pregnant teacher and plunged into some dark hole of teen angst, the male breed in particular.

Whether it was teaching English composition then or teaching running later, I found myself up against a male wall, steeped in confusing boy stuff that seemed equal parts culture and chemistry. Boys just seemed to be . . . weird. The boys I grew up with in my Brooklyn neighborhood were weird. I was weird.

I grew up with confusion over whether I should be the "good" boy or the "bad" boy—whether I should be a pacifist or aggressor, whether learning or play mattered more, whether I should pursue girls or play hard-to-get. Conflicts arose everywhere. I lost focus, had a short attention span, was erratic in school, developed fears, lacked confidence, and had no real goals other than a need to hide from responsibility.

I could easily have been one of the "classified" boys with attention deficit disorder that you hear about all the time. As an older youngster, I could have been one of the lost souls cited in the 2006 *Time* magazine article "The Trouble with Boys," who were said to be falling behind, certainly compared with girls, because of their impulsiveness, fragile ego, or plain inability to sit still.

Young males seem to be a sad lot. I was drawn to one quote in particular in the *Time* story. "Girl behavior becomes the standard. Often boys are treated like defective girls," said educator Michael Thompson, author of *Raising Cain,* a best-selling book about boys. I think that as a society we are all too ready to give up on boys, who as nongirls are framed in negative terms for almost everything they do and don't seem worth the effort.

The latest research affirms what we are beginning to realize: boys are different, not broken. In a March 2008 *New York Times Magazine* story on single-sex education ("Teaching to the Testosterone"), author Elizabeth Weil refers to educators and other experts who say that boys do not hear as well as girls and need instructors to speak louder; that boys are better at seeing action while girls see nuance and texture; that teachers need to engage boys' energy rather than inhibit it.

I wish I'd understood gender differences when I started coaching at St. Rose. After being hired, I thought: *Oh, for crying out loud . . . boys.* But I came to the task armed with good intentions, like a Peace Corps volunteer entering a third-world nation. I was not looking for "talented" runners, just boys who would try hard, because cross-country running is based on consistent training, not some natural speed afoot. I wanted to enjoy the boys— enjoy teaching them and thrilling to their successes—but I felt mired in unknown territory.

The school itself was a problem. The macho sports culture at the small, conservative Catholic school was clear. Girls who ran were admired for an endeavor that required discipline and perseverance—a pursuit considered appropriate for females, who weren't supposed to be true athletes anyway. Boys were supposed to be clashing like gladiators on the soccer field or basketball court. For them, running was the sport of last resort.

My boys brought that sense of inferiority to their running, and at first there was little I could do about it. But since cross-country required persistence and commitment from the coach as well, I decided I would work on the boys relentlessly, showering them with ideas of the value of running, how grand and exalted it was, and the noble path we could take together to contend for a state championship.

Since I knew little about boys but a fair amount about running, I realized that maybe I could learn something from them too, helping us all. If I could be more accepting of boys' supposed foibles, maybe these rascals and the naive coach could form a consonant if imperfect union, growing together toward a heaven-sent achievement.

I embarked onward for another four seasons, gaining many insights about the boys and myself, family and sharing, spirituality, and the strengths of young people confronting adversity.

THE NAME GAME

While girls tend to feel good about what they do, boys often feel good about who they are, craving an identity on which to hang their emotional hats. The most successful high school boys' cross-country coach in the nation, Joe Newton of York High in Elmhurst, Illinois, once told me that he developed crucial relationships with his runners by giving each boy a nickname, in effect a caring identity. Years later at team reunions, said Newton,

boys would come up to him, saying, "Remember me? Meathead."

No matter where you stood in the team pecking order, you
could be elevated from anonymity to recognition with a nickname. "Meathead" may not seem like a great compliment, but in
a boy's world that works. Most boys do not think of themselves as
great scholars and on a team there's nothing wrong with a little
good-natured mocking, which builds camaraderie and makes
lonely guys feel like they are "one of the boys."

Initially I had a hodgepodge of runners who were mainly trying to get in shape for other sports. The hardest worker was a
lumbering 6-foot-8-inch kid named Henry who was hoping to
gain an edge for basketball. "Big Hank," I called him. Big Hank
might have been the tallest cross-country runner in New Jersey.
As awkward a runner as Big Hank was, he completed every workout and 5K race with pride, thankful, I believe, that I chose to
single him out for his dedication.

Another endearing boy that season was Rory, who had a stride
so clean I called him "the Ethiopian," after the great runners from
that country. The nickname seemed to motivate Rory and he
would show up at practice waiting for me to say it: *Here comes
the Ethiopian.*

Bottom line: Boys need a caring identity that honors their in-
dividuality.

A WORLD APART

My second year of coaching offered a new beginning. Most of
the previous season's squad had graduated, and the newcomers
included several freshmen with no apparent history of bad habits. I tried to create a world with its own expectations to mitigate
the impact of outside forces, be they other students, the media,
or the community at large. I tried to create a family atmosphere

in which the boys would develop a sense of responsibility and commitment to one another and realize that running could be a path to self-discovery, personal growth, and maybe even a state championship.

I did this by teaching fundamentals so the boys would understand every little thing about running in order to plot their progress. I also constantly sold running as the coolest thing to do because it was arduous to run the tough hills of the cross-country course and we were like a special-forces unit on a mission only we understood for its nobility and honor. We were a Dead Poets Society for runners.

I also sought to mold this family by getting personal. From day one, at every practice and meet, I probed into each boy's personality and quirkiness, and at the same time was open about my own. I was an authority figure but not autocratic. I wanted the boys to do what they were told but contribute their own ideas. I wanted to touch each of them in a personal way, to nudge them higher, heal their wounds, and ultimately enable them to find what I felt was deep inside them: a craving to work hard, do the right thing and feel a sense of belonging, of community.

Joe Newton achieves this at York High, and he has close to 200 boys on his teams. The best cross-country coaches create a team culture that is, at its core, at odds with the outside world. If you're going to ask teenagers to run to exhaustion every day, you need to create new ways of thinking and a mountain of trust.

I tried to show my boys that I cared about them in a personal way. One student was a little guy who was self-conscious about his size and whose performances were erratic. When he tried hard, I told him he was "running with authority," which I think made him feel "bigger." That became our mantra: *You're running with authority.* At practice, he would smile when I called out the phrase, and usually pick up the pace. Another boy, Brock, was a student of running who followed the big names, thrived on routines, and like to anticipate my workouts. Eventually I referred to him as my "assistant coach" and at the start of training would say, "Okay, Brock, what's the workout for today?" Another boy took shortcuts as a way to get attention, cheating on his sit-ups or forgetting his water bottle, and I always made a point to reprimand him in a lighthearted way, giving him a long enough leash to realize that by doing right he could win attention too.

And then there was Ryan, the team's best runner, who was thoughtful and quiet, with important family issues on his mind and a tendency to burst out at a reckless pace, only to fade and perform below his capacity. He *needed* a leash on him. I would patiently admonish him, look him straight in the eye, grab him by the shoulders, give him a hug, and see if through my physical touch something of my lesson might rub off.

Bottom line: Boys need a sense of community that allows room for self-discovery.

THE REAL ME

Spending as much as five to six days a week with my boys for close to five months each season, I was very conscious of how they would regard me, what notions of maleness or manhood they would absorb from my example. From the outset, I could tell the boys gave me a good looking-over, as they would any teacher, and they would whisper about my strange habits or new haircut. In the way they would summon me by calling me, "Coach . . . ," I could also tell they wanted to know what I thought about occurrences in their lives, whether at school, at home, or in the beachfront communities in which they lived.

More than anything, I wanted the boys to feel no boundaries, challenge stereotypes, and broaden their views of appropriate male behavior. If only they would let down their guard, they would feel energized and free to relate better to teammates and myself, identify their strengths, admit weaknesses, and get closer to fulfilling their potential. Running is a mind-body-spirit endeavor, and if you were stuck on hiding your feelings or holding on to some male bitterness, you were going to have trouble conquering the cross-country course. At least that's how I felt.

So as coach, I tried to set a good example. No holding back. When they ran, I exhorted them, got animated, and embraced them at the finish, always sure to touch them with a pat on the head or rear. If someone missed practice for a silly reason, I got mad and launched into my rap on responsibility. If we had a big race and I was nervous beforehand, I showed my anxiety, confident enough that the boys would rally to the occasion instead of being dragged down by my weakness. If I made a mistake, I was quick to admit it, like the time I ridiculed a girl from another school that a boy on my team had befriended. Or the time I ordered the wrong racing strategy on a muddy course and apologized to the team afterward for our embarrassing results. If rigid school policies got in my way, I shook my head in disgust, letting them know that I felt that while the Catholic institution had many virtues, it could also suffocate ambition. In time I could laugh with them, even over their miscues, knowing their transgressions were innocent and not, as I first thought, emblematic of some great and portentous failing.

Did I really have to be the macho male adult in charge of everything, dictating, always dictating, till I was blue in the face? I knew this quote from the author Michael Thompson was true: "Boys measure everything they do or say by a single yardstick: does this make me look weak? And if it does, they're not going to do it." When I was able to let go, unconcerned about showing vulnerability, the boys could relax their own macho stance and we could all talk easily, naturally, not coach from up high to kid down below, but runner-to-runner with a feeling that we were all in this together.

They also saw me in personal crisis when my father suffered a stroke and became disabled. At practice, I would be on the phone with doctors, speaking to Dad, or feeling overwhelmed and letting tears roll down my cheeks. The boys felt for me and probably were stunned by seeing a grown man weep—their coach, no less.

At the start of my last season in the fall of 2001, when my original group of freshmen was seniors and showing the maturity to practically coach themselves, I tried in vain to fight back tears as we stood as a team in a memorial to 9/11 soon after the attack. I felt a great responsibility to ease the boys' burdens, made that much more intense by the knowledge that a team member who'd graduated the previous year had lost his father, a police officer, in the Twin Towers.

The boys had gathered silently at practice. They looked to me for guidance. I motioned for us to hold hands in a circle and suggested we pray silently, especially for John's dad. Then I sent them on their warm-up run, sat on a bench, looked out to the sea, and hoped for my boys to feel secure in their new world.

Bottom line: Boys need strong, honest, and at times vulnerable role models.

I FEEL YOUR PAIN

In my youth, I was the type of runner who played it safe, and I didn't want to convey that approach to my boys. I think I did, however. I protected them too much, and they picked up on it. Whether it was workouts or racing strategy, or merely how I engaged them in thinking about running, I probably emphasized the joy of running at the expense of hard-nosed performance. I saw how some coaches worked on their team's aggression, motivating the boys with fear. I worked on personal enrichment, steering clear of fear, which was too much for me to handle when I was a kid.

I lectured the boys on opening the mind-body door to a higher consciousness that would enable them to break through pain and defeat it, while accepting the idea that suffering was something of a spiritual quest linked to their religious education. More than anything, however, it was hard training that conquered pain, enabling a faster pace at longer distances. We did our share of tough workouts. But I rarely pushed them to the limit, never had them run longer than 6 or 7 miles, and gave them too much rest in the course of a speed workout. I babied them.

One benefit of this mistake was that it forced the boys to take some responsibility for their fitness levels. Maybe I didn't insist that they run on a Sunday or do an extra few miles before school. But a mature boy takes the initiative.

Sure enough, one day at practice my de facto assistant coach, Brock, suggested aloud that maybe we should get in more distance, more miles per week, like other teams. I thanked him but defended the nuances of our carefully calculated program. Then I thought about what he said, gathered the guys, and announced: "Brock's right. Let's do more distance."

So later that week I sent the team out on a 10-mile run. While they handled it with panache, I was so tired myself from the season and family issues that I fell asleep in my car as the boys passed me with a mile to go. Everyone enjoyed the coach's catnap and the role reversal. The boys started telling me I needed more energy if we were going to contend for a state title.

Bottom line: Boys need to be challenged to run to their limits.

A WING AND A PRAYER

The least likely runner I coached was a boy named John who wore studded jewelry, had spiked hair, created politically inspired artwork, and enjoyed challenging the school dress code. He did not belong in a parochial school and would eventually leave, mak-

ing National Honor Society in a public school and going on to
similar success in college.

But while a member of the Purple Roses, John tried as hard
as anyone, even with a tight, upright running form that made him
stand out in a crowd. In running he wanted to blend in. John got
off to a rocky start, failing to finish his first race as a freshman,
and I feared he might quit if that continued. Our team needed a
counterculture figure who could speak about geopolitics, not the
Yankees.

The rules prohibited jewelry being worn in races, and before
one meet on our home course John gave me his Catholic crucifix
to hold. I'd never held a crucifix before, but it came in handy.
During the race, as John struggled, I found myself clutching the
crucifix while reciting a Hebrew prayer of healing for John to
complete the race. Being Jewish, I'd initially been surprised that
the Catholic school had hired me, but I learned to see that as an
act of fate and used spiritual ideas where I could, like a team
prayer on the starting line, to motivate and strengthen the boys.
John finished his race, and I chalked that up to smarter pacing,
the unrelenting exhortations of the coach, and God, not necessarily in that order.

Our group prayer was a pivotal benchmark. I offered the idea
as a suggestion and the boys ran with it. Moments before each
race, a senior corralled the boys and they recited a Catholic
prayer out loud, within earshot of other teams. I felt that running
"for God" could arm the boys with faith, help unify them as a
team, and sanctify the effort. The best runners always seemed
cleansed of the drumbeat of life and able to focus on one sure
thing. By the state finals, we could too.

Being open about my Jewish identity in the Catholic environment also served my world-apart theme. The boys saw my comfort level in being different; at school functions, I was obviously
the only Jew in the room. The boys knew I would have to miss

practice for a Jewish holy day. I think they respected my commitment to my religion.

But I would not want to miss a meet, feeling the team's chances would diminish without me. When a Jewish holiday would fall on a meet date, as it seemed to every fall, I would ask the athletic director if he could change the date. He was always agreeable, and I enjoyed the idea of the athletic director of one Catholic school convincing the athletic director of another Catholic school to change a meet date for a Jewish holiday.

Bottom line: Boys need spiritual grounding for strength, faith, and commitment.

DAY OF ATONEMENT

The most memorable boys-will-be-boys incident occurred on a lovely day at the shore when I sent the team on an easy run so they'd be rested for the next day's meet. The slow pace enabled them to run together, and someone came up with the cool idea of running from the boardwalk into the ocean. In the fall, dangerous riptides develop, and when the guys dashed into the water a couple of them got caught in the surf and had to be bailed out by teammates who were lifeguards in the summer.

I waited anxiously for them. Instead of returning in fifteen minutes they came back in forty-five. They were all wet, of course, and their shoes were off. What had happened? The boys made up a story that they'd seen a man in trouble in the water and rushed in to save him. I swallowed the tale whole. (Bad example for boys: being a sucker.) That night I happened to tell a local sportswriter that my team performed an act of heroism and we arranged for a team photo on the beach the next day.

But the next morning at school the athletic director, wise to male pranks, got the real story—that a couple of my boys nearly drowned—and called me at home. I was so angry I wanted to quit. I took it personally. I felt betrayed. I told the athletic director I'd take care of it.

Between that moment and the time I got to school a few hours later, I calmed down and tried to sort out the episode and my feelings. Could anything positive come out of this? I thought of all the good things we'd experienced, how in the big picture the boys had matured, and I decided to try and make a lesson out of the incident. The punishment would be mild, but my reproach would be stern.

At school, before heading for our meet, I took the boys aside. One boy came forth with the real story and said they'd been afraid to tell me what they had done. I told the boys that the lie was worse than the deed and showed a lack of courage. They'd let me down as well as their parents and the school. And they'd let themselves down.

Then I brought up the recent Jewish holy day of Yom Kippur, the Day of Atonement for sins committed in the past year. I'd prayed for forgiveness and reminded the boys that forgiveness was a central concept in Catholic teaching. I told them that their confession was a first step toward redemption. Their punishment was that I would not hold practice for the rest of the week, and that they should run on their own; we would not compete in Saturday's statewide invitational meet; and they should write letters of apology to the athletic director and the newspaper that had planned the feature story.

I could tell they were sorry for what they done, ashamed that male impulses had led them astray. I hoped I was now teaching them a lesson that the male tendency toward vengeance was not the only path toward reconciliation. Maybe I was bringing them back to their church.

The next day I received an e-mail apology from the team that concluded with these words: "We will try to regain your trust by our future actions and hope that we can make you proud." And indeed they would.

   Bottom line: Boys need to know that forgiveness and reconciliation can resolve conflict.

WINNING PARENTS

I had no problem with the type of overbearing parents who meddle with their kids' sports teams. From the outset I embraced parents with an open-arms strategy to engage them, instruct them, and try to win their trust. It seemed to work.

   Working in my favor was that parents of boys tend to be less proactive and in your face than parents of girls, many of whom feel a need to "protect" their young and may take issue with team pecking order, perceived slights, and exactly how the coach addresses their daughter. Parents of boys tend to take either a laissez-faire approach or let you know their son is a rascal and needs a kick in the pants every so often. I decided that our parents could be an asset in helping to develop the boys' commitment. If they could see their sons' gains, they would get behind my program and go to the mat for me.

   At every practice, I stuck my head into the car windows of parents picking up their kids and told them how their sons were doing, emphasizing the positive while not shying away from the negative. I was never punitive in tone; all goals centered on learning and my crusade to use running as a wellspring of conviction for the boys. I called homes regularly in the evenings to report on progress, great practices, negligence, and non-running-related issues that I thought parents should know about. Parents, in turn, would call me to say how their son was doing, or to ask if maybe I could speak with Johnny because his grades were suffering or he was hanging out with the wrong crowd.

Parents saw that I cared about their sons. Whether as helpers at meets or in rallying their sons to leap onto my bandwagon, parents would function as assistant coaches. Not once did any parent lobby for his son to receive any sort of recognition; if anything, they gave me a free hand in disciplining their kids, in situations like the ocean episode. We were a team.

In November 2000, every team parent turned out for support as we attempted to win the school's first state Parochial B title in twelve years. Would Ryan rise above personal issues and run the race he could? Would Justin, recently injured, find the strength to fulfill his critical team role? Both boys performed to their potential, running their best races. Indeed, every boy ran his best and we were victorious. But what made me proudest on the day we won our first state title was the humility the boys showed in accepting their honors. The key runners on the squad were all juniors, and they returned to repeat their championship run in 2001.

Bottom line: Boys need involved parents to support the coach and team.

9

Running with Teen Dreams

I can hardly think of a kid on our squad who has missed a race because of injury or illness. We stress moderation and consistency. We want to be stronger with each day and each year.

—Dan Fitzsimmons, state championship
high school coach in South Dakota

For young runners, the teenage years present important changes in age, socialization, physical and emotional development, maturity, and competitive opportunity. I saw it myself with my own children and as well with the high school team that I coached. When my two daughters started running high school track and cross-country as 14-year-old freshmen, they lacked focus, had no goals, took little initiative, and resisted my attempts to help them improve. I could chalk that up to immaturity, teen angst, or not wanting a know-it-all dad dictating the terms of engagement. By junior and senior years, they didn't need my guidance. The girls were hardworking team leaders moving up in the ranks of successful runners.

The freshman boys who came out for my cross-country team could barely tie their running shoes properly without help. But by junior and senior years the boys were teaching me a few things, and our team's maturity led to a pair of state championships.

In many ways, youngsters enter high school as children and come out as adults. They may start out physically as tiny little things and finish as big, strong, aggressive athletes. They may be shy and tentative at first and eventually become polished role models who help set a team's tone, on and off the running course. Even youngsters who begin running in grade school enter a new and threatening world in high school as they confront the myriad teen issues of peer acceptance. As intimidating as a new team can be, a team can also offer a comfortable entree into high school, as runners tend to be welcoming, no one gets cut from cross-country or track, and there are many introductory races to nurture young talent. I have had many top high school runners, girls and boys, tell me how freshman cross-country got them off to a pivotal start in high school, not only as runners but as impressionable young people trying to cope with the high school maelstrom.

One was Ben Johnson, a state champion in track and cross-country and a nationally ranked runner at New Mexico's Albuquerque Academy in 2007 and 2008. Johnson traced his success to his freshman season, when he tagged along with older teammates training in the rain on challenging mountain paths. Even though he was initiated with some mud-splattering, Benjo (as his coach started calling him) saw a work ethic that appealed to him, made friends right away, and felt at ease in the older crowd. He also saw sensitivity. That first season the coach had undergone surgery and was recuperating at home. The team members decided to do a symbolic run to the coach's home to offer their support. Benjo said, "I saw all the caring on the team and wanted to be a part of that."

HIGH SCHOOL TEAMS NURTURE ALL LEVELS

Most high school teams offer similar encouragement. Track and cross-country can be very competitive, but you rarely find the kind of winning-is-everything attitude evident in some other sports. Even in high-powered programs noted for their trophy collections, there are many levels of emphasis, from novice to national level, and ready acceptance of all abilities, needs, goals, and personalities. The York High School boys of Elmhurst, Illinois, have won a record twenty-six state cross-country titles, but only some of the squad's 175 youngsters do the bare-knuckles training programs that contribute to such success. The majority of coach Joe Newton's youngsters join the team to get in shape, make friends, and have a school identity. They're looking for personal records, not state records.

That is the wonderful thing about high school running: you set your own agenda. There are no soccer goals or basketball minutes or football catches or gymnastics scores to be judged by. In running, you can't help improving almost every time out. And if you're lucky enough to join a good team with a caring, knowledgeable coach, success and enjoyment can be boundless.

Take two girls who live near me in New Jersey, Ashley Higginson and Rachel Morris. My wife, Andrea, is a second-grade teacher in the local district, and both Ashley and Rachel were students in her class, so I took an interest in their progress. Ashley ran for Colts Neck High and as a freshman was not a star by any means. However, under the patient tutelage of coach Jim Schlentz, Ashley improved year by year, becoming a three-time national champion in track and cross-country as a senior. She was also an outstanding student and is now starring at Princeton University.

Rachel, two years younger than Ashley, started jogging with her father at an early age. I would see her at local races and give her advice. She was the type of kid who wanted to run longer and longer, 5 miles and up as she approached high school. Rachel also attended Colts Neck, loved track and cross-country, and by junior year worked her way onto the varsity cross-country unit, scoring key points in the state meet. Shy and reserved before high school, Rachel blossomed on the team and at this writing more improvement awaited her in senior year. She also hopes to run in college.

PATIENCE IS THE COACH'S MANTRA

Higginson has said many times that as a coach, Schlentz "makes you love running." His secret? He holds you back. Patience is his mantra. One summer day in 2006 when I visited his team practice on the hilly state cross-country course, Schlentz, who's been coaching for thirty years, was explaining the process to the younger runners. In effect, it was a plea. He could tell they wanted to follow the pace set by the team's older runners. "If I let you run hard, you'll just survive," Schlentz told them. "Build each mile. Learn to feel good."

The workout that evening was a series of mile runs at a crisp pace, separated by a brief rest, on the hilly terrain. When the athletes were finished and glowing with accomplishment, Schlentz turned to me and said, "You have to keep them hungry. You want these kids running great as juniors and seniors because you haven't pounded them. That's the key."

Indeed it is. Let Schlentz's mantra be your guide. Whether you're male or female, new to running or experienced, hoping just to get in shape and make friends or become a champion, part of an average team or state contender, be patient. Resist the temptation, seen throughout youth sports, to excel as soon as possible, as though your body clock is ticking. Replace "ASAP" with "BPAT" (be patient and thrive). Here's how patience and good sense can be applied to all aspects of high school running.

JOIN THE HIGH SCHOOL TEAM

You can enjoy running on your own, but the high school team is really a necessity for learning, improvement, sharing the hard work of running with friends, and the opportunity to compete in many exciting track and cross-country meets. "Running on the high school team," wrote former New York State cross-country champion Brian Dalpiaz in the *Runner's World* high school magazine, "improves social skills and helps you relate better to everyone."

Cross-country is a fall sport with summer training that for most schools begins in June or July. Track and field is a spring sport with a winter indoor track season in about half the states. In states without indoor track, athletes either train through the winter or participate in other sports. Many athletes run year-round, which has both benefits and drawbacks. I advise newer runners to take one season off, usually the winter, to get a break from running; some young athletes play soccer in the fall for a couple of years, then run track in spring. Soccer is excellent conditioning for running (see "Diversify Your Sports Program" later in this chapter).

TRACK YOUR PROGRESS

It's essential to keep a running diary or scrapbook to track your progress and serve as motivation. Record training, racing, goals, assessments from yourself and what the coach says, your feelings about running, inspirational sayings you pick up, even eating habits. You might find that having a big breakfast is best before races, or discover that eating lightly works for you. In training, it's helpful to see what you've accomplished and where you're going.

No runner can keep all this information in his head. A day-by-day chronology also fosters a patient approach, as you can chart any indication of progress, affirming that a deliberate approach is working. Plus, you find extra motivation in reviewing your best workouts, where you make breakthroughs, and the instances when the coach gave you an extra pat on the back.

Obviously, you can keep all this in a computer file, but some runners still prefer doing it the old-fashioned way with a big notebook or loose-leaf binder. Runners like to be able to throw their diaries into their track bag to read on the bus to a meet, or bring it to practice on occasion to share with teammates. The running diary is a testament to success, something to treasure for years to come.

Your diary can also be a tool for coaches. At Jesuit High in Portland, Oregon, coach Tom Rothenberger checks athlete diaries for training patterns and for reflective comments that indicate an athlete's mindset and any potential problems.

BE COACHABLE

One of the biggest compliments you can receive as an athlete is that you're very "coachable." That means you cooperate with the coach, follow instructions, show initiative, help teammates, volunteer for extra tasks, and value learning at all times. In other words, you're a good student. You follow training rules, always have the proper gear, come to practice and meets on time, and let the coach know if you have any problems or feel ready for accelerated running perhaps earlier than scheduled. Being coachable also means asking constructive questions, for example, about which events you should enter at meets, or teams you're competing against, or maybe questioning the coach about information of interest to your parents. A coachable athlete does not follow blindly; he or she thinks and, when appropriate, asks questions.

A coachable athlete is also sensitive to the job a coach has in supervising a large group of athletes on a tight schedule. The coach is not always available to give every team member personal attention. Some of that attention may have to be given via e-mail. Some track and cross-country teams have upward of 50 or even 100 or more members. The head coach may have one or more assistant coaches, or may manage the team himself. Gradually acquire a sense of how the team operates, and learn the best times to address the coach with personal matters.

A FOUR-YEAR DISTANCE PLAN

If you did nothing but long, slow distance training for four years of high school, you would gain tremendous fitness, develop high aerobic capacity, and steadily improve your racing performances year by year. High school distance success, in the 1,600 meters and 3,200 meters in track (or 1 mile and 2 mile) and 5,000-meter (5K) event in cross-country, is based primarily on a steady volume of comfortably paced running week after week and month after month. Even Olympic-level runners often do several months of distance before launching into high-gear "quality" training.

Distance is the key, the foundation, what's often called your "base." As you get older and stronger and gain experience, you can increase the amount of running you do every week. A gradual climb in weekly mileage over a four-year period can take you from novice to junior varsity to varsity and beyond. Consistent mileage trumps everything, including talent, which applies more to sprints and power events than distance. How do you ensure a consistent mileage increase? With modest increases; remember, no rushing. The more you rush, the greater the risk of injury. With every injury, you take a step backward—a giant step backward in the case of something severe like a stress fracture, which typically requires several weeks' layoff.

People like to say that "injuries are part of running." Why join the crowd? Even if you're ambitious and hope to be running as much as 70 miles a week, 10 miles a day, by senior year—an elite level—by starting modestly as a freshman with 15 or 20 miles a week, you'll have more than enough time to reach your mileage goal. Gradually increase mileage as you get older and stronger and your body grows.

Many excellent high school runners finish their four years at 35 or 40 miles a week. Sure, some do 80 or even 100. Olympic marathoner Dathan Ritzenhein ran up to 95 miles a week in high school in Michigan. However, American 5,000-meter record holder Bob Kennedy did 40 or so in high school in Ohio. World championship 10,000-meter bronze medalist Kara Goucher trained 35 a week in high school in Minnesota. Two-time NCAA 10,000 titlist Alicia Shay ran up to 70 a week in high school in Wyoming.

As you can tell, there's no one "best" mileage plan. Some runners handle higher mileage better than others. By progressing gradually, you'll learn what you can tolerate (keep reviewing that diary) and be able to make adjustments with minimal injury risk. This long-term approach is used successfully at South Dakota's Yankton High, whose girls' cross-country team has been high in the national rankings the past five years. In a fall 2006 interview, coach Dan Fitzsimmons told me, "I can hardly think of a kid on our squad who has missed a race because of injury or illness. We stress moderation and consistency. We want to be stronger with each day and each year."

SEPARATE BUT EQUAL

Girls and boys run the same events in track and cross-country with one exception: in about a dozen states the girls' official cross-country distance remains less than 5K, either 2 miles (as in Texas) or 4K (as in Iowa). Even in these states, some invitational meets have 5K races for girls, who also get to run 5K when their schools travel to other states for competition. So for the most part girls don't really lose out.

In track, the most recent distance event added for girls is the steeplechase, held in only a handful of states for both boys and girls. Boys run the 3,000-meter steeple (the international standard) while girls usually run a 2,000-meter steeple. It's a token difference.

By and large, boys and girls can do the same training year-round. Because of adolescent growth differences, girls should be extra careful to train modestly prior to the onset of puberty (see chapter 7). Coaches who work with both boys and girls teams typically dish out the same workouts to both squads, but girls may end up doing less mileage. If, for example, a coach has his athletes run for an hour, girls will tend to run less distance since their pace on average would be a little slower.

Coach Fitzsimmons of South Dakota, who coaches boys and girls, said he picked up an important gender distinction from Villanova coach Marcus O'Sullivan, the former world-class miler. Because boys are more heavily muscled than girls, their muscles break down more readily from interval running, affecting their race times. When Fitzsimmons slowed the pace of boys' intervals (while shortening the rest period to maintain intensity), he found their race times "dropping like crazy."

WELCOME TOUGH CONDITIONS

Three-time world cross-country champion and Olympic 10,000-meter bronze medalist Lynn Jennings always said that the worse the conditions, the better she ran. Jennings won several of her thirty-eight U.S. national titles in rain, snow, and freezing temperatures. When it comes to bad weather, you can complain about it, make excuses, and lower your goals or do as

Jennings did—think positively and use the challenge as an advantage over your opposition.

Every fall season at Nike Cross Nationals in Portland, Oregon, the premier high school cross-country meet of the year, race conditions are demanding: rain, snow flurries, temperatures in the 30s, and a muddy course. But most of the field does not think, *That's horrible.* They think, *It's an opportunity to show toughness—and what fun it is to run in the mud.* It's that attitude that vaulted the athletes and their teams to national standing in the first place.

You don't even need experience in tough conditions to thrive, just a good head. The 2007 Nike Cross Nationals individual winners were Chris Derrick of Illinois, who was used to flat, dry courses, and Madeline Morgan of Alabama, who typically ran in the sun. "I'm definitely not a mudder," said Derrick. "I haven't seen snow in seven years," said Morgan. But they won.

BE A GOOD TEAMMATE

Cross-country is first and foremost a team sport, and coaches preach team running in which athletes stick together in practice and races, making one another that much stronger. Studies have shown that runners feel less fatigue in group efforts, and there's extra motivation in holding a good pace with teammates in tow. Distance runners have a natural tendency to support one another. Even rivals from different teams usually embrace one another after a tough race. There's a shared spirit that lifts all runners, and if you have a disappointing race or personal problem, chances are that teammates will come to your aid.

This approach dictates the pulse of the Fayetteville-Manlius girls of New York, national team cross-country champions in 2006 and 2007. In their undefeated fall '07 campaign, five different girls were the team's number-one runners at various times, as the expected top performer nursed a season-long ankle injury. "None of them cares who the first runner is," said coach Bill Aris that fall. He said that at their best the girls blended as one, and their racing showed that. At Nike Cross Nationals '07, the top four Hornets girls finished within 24 seconds, an enviably tight team spread in the 5K event, and the fifth finisher, the girl with the ankle problem, was only another 28 seconds back.

While track and field tends to emphasize individual achievement, good teammates are still essential, especially with regard to relays. At the 2005 high school nationals in Greensboro, North Carolina, Aislinn Ryan of New York's Warwick Valley High could not do enough for teammates after anchoring the distance medley relay to fourth place in an emotional climax to the spring season. Ryan, the 2004 Foot Locker national cross-country champion, had another year of high school to go, but her relay mates were all seniors sitting in tears after their last high school race. Ryan came to their aid with hugs, a water bottle, and comforting words with a nurse's bedside manner.

"I love those girls like my sisters," said Ryan, now competing for Colorado University.

"That's Aislinn," said Warwick girls coach Richard Furst at the time. "Always thinking about the team. I've got young girls who want to be her teammate, to wrap around her." Be a good teammate. Be like Aislinn.

USE TRAINING VARIETY

In addition to distance runs, there are four other primary training methods to get you in peak shape: hill running, tempo runs, long intervals (or repetitions), and short intervals. These methods enrich training by adding intensity, with the goal of improving performance for competition. In addition, every runner likes variety. Coaches know this and have countless ways of setting up training for a week, month, and entire season—and as part of a four-year plan.

Hills

Running hills, especially for cross-country, works the aerobic system and muscles at a high level but without pounding the body as you would on a track or the roads. You can run hilly courses, like the Los Alamos team in New Mexico does on the high mountain trails surrounding the school. Or you can do hill sprints, recommended by professional coach Brad Hudson, who has national champions like Dathan Ritzenhein and Jorge Torres run 10 seconds all-out on a steep hill and repeat that several times for high-octane power. Or you can do something like a dozen runs of a gently sloping 250-meter hill, a favorite workout of 2005 Foot Locker national runner-up Andrew Bumbalough of Tennessee, who now runs for Georgetown.

Whatever your workout, be aware of correct running form on hills, where your body position changes. Says Jim Schlentz, the New Jersey coach: (1) shorten your stride, (2) move your arms up and back (not side to side) with elbows high, (3) keep your back straight with a slight forward lean, not letting your torso droop, and (4) look straight ahead, not looking down, or your shoulders and neck will tighten. Some runners find going downhill harder than uphill. "Running downhill," advises Schlentz, "lengthen your stride and lower your knees, keeping your hips under you and shoulders slightly in front of you. Don't lean back in a 'braking' motion; that will only slow you down."

Tempo Runs

These are short distance runs at a brisk pace, roughly 30–45 seconds slower than 5K race pace, about 80 percent of maximum effort. If you run the 5K at 6 minutes per mile, then a 3-to-5-mile run at about 6:30 to 6:45 per mile is a tempo workout. These workouts, sometimes called lactate threshold runs, raise your anaerobic threshold, the point at which leg-tiring lactic acid will build up in the muscle.

Long Intervals

These efforts—repeated runs of 800 meters, 1,000 meters, or a mile at a fast pace—are bread-and-butter workouts that tax your system to the max. They can be done on grass, track, or the roads, and may feel harder than an actual race. That's the point: to give you strength and what some coaches call "callusing" for competition. Professional coach Joe Vigil, who has worked with Olympic marathon medalist Deena Kastor and other stars, recommends a weekly session of 5 × 1,000 meters for high school cross-country. Coach Jeff Arbogast of Bingham High in Utah, whose girls' team has been ranked number one in the country, uses 6 × 800 meters as a staple. The three-time New York City Marathon champion Alberto Salazar, a professional coach who has also worked with high school athletes, finds mixing the distance and surface inspires his runners. He advises a fast 800 on the track, then 3 × 1,200 meters uphill on the road, finishing with another 800 on the track.

Short Intervals

Speed work, like repeat 200s and 400s, in which you run faster than race pace, is usually saved for late in the season for sharpening up and working on leg turnover, so your body can move smoothly at a high rate of speed. Dan Fitzsimmons, the South Dakota coach, reserves intervals, from 200 to 1,000, for the last three weeks of the season. At Omaha Marian High, seven-time Nebraska state girls cross-country champion, coach Roger Wright uses the midseason for weekly 200s, then has his team taper off in the last couple of weeks before state.

BECOME A CROSS-TRAINER

There's a hardly a runner anywhere, from high school to college to the pros, who doesn't cross-train with nonimpact exercise such as swimming, water running, bicycling, or the elliptical machine for excellent conditioning while giving the body a break from the pounding of running. Cross-training reduces injury risk, and it helps you recover if you are hurt. World-class runner Lauren Fleshman has included some bicycling in her recent development. The Princeton University women's team uses pool work as often as three times a week. The University of Michigan women rely on the elliptical machine for a full-body, nonrunning workout. Tennessee high school star Sean Keveran of Brentwood High did several weeks of pool training in the winter of 2007, his junior year, because of an injury, and says that approach refreshed him for the spring, when he had a track breakthrough, running a nationally ranked time for 2 miles.

STRETCH IT OUT

There are many views of stretching, but the consensus is that you should warm up the body first with 5 or 10 minutes of easy running before stretching, and stretching should consist of a combination of static stretches (holding a stretch in one position) and dynamic stretches (moving the body through a range of motion), done both before and after the workout. Every team has its own style, usually based on coaching trial and error.

▶ The Spence Family on Enjoying Running

Neely Spence, the 2008 national high school girls' 2-mile champion, joins younger running sisters Margeaux and Reynah in offering ideas on young runners. Their father, Steve Spence, was the world championship bronze medalist in the marathon in 1991 and is track and cross-country coach at Shippensburg University in Pennsylvania, where Neely began college in the fall of 2008.

Their suggestions: Kids can start running at any age, but before age 12 extreme care should be taken with the amount of running they do. Running should be handled on the child's terms. The idea of going for a run should be child-initiated and a parent should accompany the child. A run around the neighborhood, to a friend's house or to an ice cream shop sounds good. Competition should be at the participatory level and only once or twice a year.

After 12, running more regularly, say, three or four times a week, is recommended. Parents can encourage running, but it still needs to be based on fun and done with friends or family. Racing can be participatory or start to become competitive and should be limited to one or two races a month, and not year-round. Competition should be team-oriented, promoting leadership skills. It needs to be grounded in sportsmanship and teach life lessons like goal setting, working as a group to achieve common goals, finding your individual niche, and being positive in the face of adversity. These values are more important than winning or personal bests.

We have found that the running experience has turn-ons and turn-offs. Turn-ons include the freedom and independence that come from doing a sport that's totally about you and your body and the elements that day, and the feeling of accomplishment that running gives you. Turn-offs include when parents lose the process orientation of our sport and become goal-driven toward their children's achievements.

At Delaware state girls champion Tatnall High, coach Pat Castagno has a favorite stretch he calls "scorpions," done like this with fifteen repeats on each side: (1) lie on your chest in a star pattern, legs spread slightly greater than shoulder width and arms perpendicular to the body, palms down; (2) swing one leg across the back side of the body to try to touch the opposite hand, then back to start position; (3) do the same motion with the other leg. Keep the legs in constant movement to work the body through a full range of motion. "This is excellent for the front-side hip flexors and external obliques [trunk rotation muscles]," says Castagno, pointing out that tight hip flexors commonly cause injury.

GET SOME MUSCLE

Weight training specific to running strengthens you for racing and helps prevent injury. Indiana state girls' titlist Westfield High is in the weight room two to three times a week year-round. "A stronger upper body means better arm carry and less 'cross center,' taking stress off the lower body," says coach Scott Lidskin. "We bench-press with the goal of reaching 85 percent or more of weight by end of junior year." All of the varsity cross-country runners achieve that. They also do core body work including push-ups.

Core exercise (working the abdominals and back) was also at the heart of the South Lakes High program in Virginia that produced high school mile record breaker Alan Webb, now a top pro. As at Westfield, Webb's coach, Scott Raczko, had the runners in the weight room all year, using mostly free weights for all muscle groups while emphasizing the core. "You have to be strong," says Raczko, "so your form does not break down late in a race."

At New York City Catholic school Monsignor Farrell of Staten Island, an all-boys school with a 100-man squad, coach Tom

Cuffe orders twice-weekly weight work with machines and free weights that includes running in place while holding light dumbbells, moving the arms up and back through the "power zone." Says Cuffe: "Arms generate power. Power equals speed. That's the essence of running."

FIX FORM FLAWS

Some people say not to mess with a runner's natural form, but Jim Schlentz, the New Jersey coach, is a stickler for the three Fs—fix form flaws—and has seen the benefits in his champion athletes. Schlentz maintains that by relaxing the arms and shoulders, "opening the chest," you breathe in more air and have more oxygen for the muscles. This also leads to a smoother stride and less energy expenditure for a given effort. Schlentz' pointers: (1) swing your arms low, at the waist, to prevent knees from rising too high, resulting in overstriding; (2) move your arms up and back with elbows at a 90-degree angle, for faster leg movement; (3) keep shoulders relaxed, so the entire body is relaxed and flowing; and (4) keep shoulders "quiet," as opposed to turning them back and forth, which wastes energy and brings hands inward, hindering breathing.

Another way to prevent overstriding is to count strides per minute, a remedy at New York's Hilton High in the Rochester area, 2005 national girls' cross-country champion. Using studies by the noted coach and exercise physiologist Jack Daniels, Hilton coach Mike Szczepanik looks for a count of at least 90 strides per minute (counting one leg). Szczepanik says that runners with lower counts, say, around 80, tend to get more injuries because they're "in the air longer," overstriding, and strike the ground harder with each stride.

WORK ON MIND POWER

Coaches increasingly recognize the power of the mind, and the
mental training slogans on running T-shirts attest to that.
Whether at practice or prior to competition, athletes find inner
strength in various ways. One trend seems to be a preference toward being psyched "down" rather than psyched "up." Utah state
champion Luke Puskedra of Judge Memorial says, "I like to practice yoga to get everything in tune." New York State champion
Pat Dupont of Fairport says, "I don't try to get psyched up. I try to
relax by falling into old habits." Foot Locker girls' 2006 national
runner-up Aurora Scott of Virginia says, "Relax, relax, relax. Practice relaxing."

The Connecticut state champion Danbury High boys' team
puts relaxation to the ultimate test. Before a race, if any athlete is
stressed, coach Rob Murray has him lie on the ground and relax
moments before the gun sounds. To opponents, that approach
might look like a sign of weakness, but to Murray it enhances
positive mental attitude. Prior to meets, the team works on
breathing, visualization, and staying in the moment. "I also give
the boys affirmations," said Murray, "that I say aloud and ask
them to repeat to themselves. For example, 'I am prepared to fulfill my potential.'"

DIVERSIFY YOUR SPORTS PROGRAM

There's nothing wrong with running cross-country and track year-
round for four years, but virtually nonstop running can increase
injury risk, get tedious at times, prevent you from enjoying other
sports, and limit your overall experience as a growing teen. In
states with little or no indoor track, runners may swim or play
basketball in the winter. In the New York–New Jersey area, where
indoor track is very big with weekly meets at the Armory Track

and Field Center in Manhattan, many cross-country runners barely catch their breath after the fall season before jumping into track. Some of these youngsters are best served with a low-key indoor campaign, doing relays, trying new events, and getting in some cross-training.

Oftentimes, multiple sports issues revolve around soccer, typically a fall sport like cross-country. Young athletes who come to high school with a soccer background—and these days, who doesn't?—start out on the school soccer team (sometimes also playing on community and traveling teams), demonstrate running ability, and within a year or two face the decision of whether to switch to cross-country. This switch has produced countless success stories. In my area of New Jersey, to cite one example, twins Katy and Amanda Trotter of Red Bank Regional played soccer in their freshman, sophomore, and junior fall seasons while running track in winter and spring; they switched to cross-country as seniors and placed one-two in the state meet. They went on to run at Stanford.

However, because of soccer pressures—coach or family not wanting to let go—some youngsters try to do soccer and cross-country simultaneously. It may be too much. "Last year," says Andrew Hudson, coach of 2007 Georgia state girls' cross-country champion Collins Hill, "we had one runner whose performances worsened because of her overbearing soccer schedule. Twice a week she was going from cross-country practice to two-hour soccer practices, and then on weekends she had soccer matches after meets. We told her that two sports were hurting her running but that it was her decision. Finally, she quit soccer, got her energy back, and helped us win the state meet."

▶ High School Runner (and Parent) Bill of Rights

Track and cross-country athletes and their parents should have certain rights to protect their interests and enhance their experience. These are meant as guidelines and may vary somewhat with the school, team, or community.

Runners' Bill of Rights

1. To be team members in good standing as long as they attend practice and behave properly based on the coach's policies.

2. To not be cut from the team based on performance.

3. To be treated equally with all team members regardless of performance.

4. To be spoken to with respect and decency by the coach, other team members, and school officials.

5. To be given proper training methods based on age and experience.

6. To compete in events appropriate to age, experience, and ability.

7. To have proper gear and instruction to facilitate efforts safely.

8. To be given sufficient rest in order to recover from rigorous training and competition.

9. To not be forced to diet or lose weight to meet any standards.

10. To have privacy safeguarded in locker rooms.

11. To have safe transport to meets and other venues.

12. To be able to compete in postseason events as they choose.

13. To be given proper care when hurt or injured.

14. To be given proper care in emergency health situations.

15. To be told eligibility rules in advance so that policies are understood.

16. To have some input into which events they compete in.

17. To be able to drink water, etc., as needed at practice.

18. To be able to speak with the coach about any problems like training difficulties or conflicts with teammates.

Parents' Bill of Rights

1. To be able to communicate with the coach on a regular basis.

2. To know what is expected of the athlete during the season.

3. To know the practice schedule from day to day.

4. To know the meet schedule and transportation system.

5. To be informed of any problem regarding the athlete.

6. To be updated on the athlete's progress.

7. To attend meets and watch the athlete compete.

8. To know what gear is necessary and any costs involved.

9. To know safety precautions when the team travels.

10. To know procedures if the athlete incurs an injury.

11. To know procedures in a medical emergency.

12. To know broadly how athletes are trained and whether prolonged fatigue or soreness can be expected.

13. To be able to view team practice on occasion.

14. To be informed of any major out-of-pocket costs in advance.

15. To know if girls or boys on the same squad are handled any differently, and for what reasons.

16. To know if the athlete has special talent and what opportunities that may present.

17. To be informed of any sudden change in the athlete's behavior or attitude.

18. To be assured that the athlete will not be placed in compromising situations traveling with adult personnel.

▶ **Should Teens Run Marathons?**

Not every high school runner participates on a school team. There is a growing movement, especially in urban areas, for privately run organizations to partner with schools and promote teenage running programs based on completing a half-marathon or marathon. Is running 26.2 miles too much of a good thing for kids?

Every March, more than 2,000 middle school and high school youngsters, ages twelve to eighteen, run the City of Los Angeles Marathon. (Beginning in 2009, the event will be run on Memorial Day.) Called Students Run LA, it's a growing program in its twentieth year, geared primarily to at-risk inner-city youth. The students get medical clearance, train for months with volunteer coaches at 150 schools, and must complete an 18-mile time trial to prove readiness. "The kids gain health and maturity, and finishing the marathon has a ripple effect," said one of the program's creators, Paul Trapani, a teacher. The marathoners' high school graduation rate is 90 percent in an area where the norm is about 60 percent. Trapani also points to the remarkable finishing rate, as high as 99 percent, higher than that for adults in the race.

Despite such findings, many sports medicine experts like Dr. Stephen G. Rice, director of the Jersey Shore Sports Medicine Center at University Medical Center in Neptune, New Jersey, argue against young marathoners. In a 2003 article in the *Clinical Journal of Sports Medicine*, Rice wrote that the combination of kids' growing musculoskeletal system and the repetitive trauma of running for an extended period of time increased youngsters' risk of injury. "Why push the envelope?" Rice told me in an interview. "Kids can run 5Ks and 10Ks." This view is consistent with policy statements of the American Academy of Pediatrics.

Other dissenters include Dr. Lyle Michaeli, director of sports medicine at Children's Hospital Boston, whose negative view led the Boston Marathon to adopt an age requirement of eighteen. "When a youngster's body is still growing," says Boston race director Guy Morse, "then the strain of the marathon is magnified. Play it safe. There's no need to rush it."

On the Run: A Primer for Ages 15 to 18

Starting out. With cross-country in the fall and track in the winter (in most states) and spring, plus summer training, running can become a year-round endeavor for the full four years of high school. Take a patient approach, trying to improve a little each season, with the idea of learning from the coach and older athletes and moving up in the team standings. Establish goals for each season and be prepared to alter those goals as you develop.

Healthy fun. To reduce injury risk, it's good strategy to take one season off from running and do another sport, at least for the first year or two. Even top runners benefit from that approach. The strength and fitness from other sports, such as soccer, basketball, swimming, or gymnastics, can be beneficial in running.

Must-do stretches. High school coaches increasingly emphasize core exercises in which you strengthen the body's midsection—the abdominals, hips, and lower back. Aside from regular team practice, do sit-ups and crunches on your own and use a medicine ball and other devices for a range of exercises that build core strength. There are numerous Web sites with advice and products.

Fail-safe workouts. Team practice is usually Monday through Friday with meets on Saturday, and sometimes during the week. Coaches often require, or encourage, a long Sunday run on your own or with teammates at a comfortable pace. Make sure you

(continued)

don't skimp on that. Connect with teammates and start out with a goal of 45 minutes to an hour, increasing time with each year so you reach 90 minutes or more as a senior. This is a great strength builder.

Helpful parents. Parents can help by assisting the coach with clerical or other duties at home meets, getting involved in fundraising for team travel, and hosting pre-event pasta dinners that are a staple of many programs. Encourage youngsters to enjoy all aspects of the team experience so they don't use race performance as the only source of satisfaction.

Running distances. Cross-country races are 3 miles or 5K (3.1 miles) for boys and 2 miles, 4K (2.5 miles), 3 miles, or 5K (3.1 miles) for girls, depending on state rules. Track distances run from the sprints to 3,200 meters or 2 miles with some 5K events in national meets. Freshman cross-country is usually about 1.5 to 2 miles. Here are some suggestions for various ages:

School Year (Age)	Frequency
Freshman (15)	Daily practice, take one season off for other sports
Sophomore (16)	Daily practice, take one season off for other sports
Junior (17)	Daily practice, running year-round
Senior (18)	Daily practice, running year-round

School Year (Age)	Miles Per Week
Freshman (15)	Up to 20 miles a week
Sophomore (16)	20 to 30 miles a week
Junior (17)	30 to 40 miles a week
Senior (18)	40 miles a week and up

Racing by age. Suggested race distances for high schoolers:

School Year (Age)	Race Distance
Freshman (15)	Sprints to 2 miles
Sophomore (16)	Sprints to 5K (3.1 miles)
Junior (17)	Sprints to 5K (3.1 miles)
Senior (18)	Sprints to 5K (3.1 miles), or 10K (6.2 miles) in off-season

Target mile times. These provide safe, comfortable goals.

Age	Boys' Target	Girls' Target
Freshman (15)	5:15	6:00
Sophomore (16)	5:00	5:45
Junior (17)	4:45	5:30
Senior (18)	4:30	5:15

(For boys 4:20 or better is elite level; for girls, it's 5:05 or better.)

10

Running with Danny

I'd point out things like deer, horses. When Danny would say "horses" to me, I knew he wanted to run the reservoir route.

—PAT MANTONE, DANNY'S TEACHER, COACH,
AND RUNNING GURU IN NEW JERSEY

It's a breathtaking fall day as young runners gather for their first league cross-country meet of the season on the grounds of Marlboro Middle School in central New Jersey. The sun is out, the temperature balmy, and the winds light as Danny Mininsohn, a 12-year-old seventh grader at the host school, waits to run with his 100-plus teammates against the competition from Marlboro Memorial and Eisenhower Middle School of Freehold Township.

"How do you manage the course for someone like Danny?" says his mom, Anne Marie, to no one in particular.

"I'm a nervous wreck," says Anne Marie's sister, Danny's aunt Kathy, who sometimes picks up Danny after school.

Danny stands a hair under five feet, weighs 100 pounds and has the bony trimness of an endurance athlete. He wears the royal blue racing colors of Marlboro Middle and a red headband purchased by his grandmother, Anne Marie's mom, so he can be spotted from a distance on the cross-country course. He also wears a new pair of customized New Balance trail shoes purchased at a shop catering to people with special needs.

"Those shoes are so cool," says the Marlboro Middle boys' cross-country coach, Caolan Sinisi, 27, a special-education teacher and avid runner herself. When I coached at St. Rose, Caolan's twin sisters were members of the school's girls' squad. She is the oldest of five girls, all with blazing red hair and sweet dispositions. When I tell her of my interest in Danny, Caolan says, "I feel like crying."

"I'm so excited that the coach has knowledge of autism," says Anne Marie. "Everything is aligned in the right way. Like the coach said, Danny deserves to be here. He ran all summer. I'm looking for an indoor track for the winter."

Team Danny huddles near the start as Danny prepares to join his team for prerace stretching exercises. Everyone is present: family, friends, and teachers, including his special-education teacher, Sue Webster, and the elementary school PE teacher who got Danny started running and nurtures him like family: Pat Mantone.

When someone in the group calls out that Danny has big feet, Danny repeats, "Big feet, big feet . . ."

Danny takes his seated position in a big circle with the team as Sinisi supervises stretching, each movement held to a count of ten. Danny is able to mimic simple exercises like toe touches. When he has trouble with more complex movements, he is assisted by a teammate, Nick, who repositions Danny's legs correctly. "Nick keeps an eye on Danny when he's running," says Anne Marie.

Sinisi reviews the course, which the team has run in practice. It consists of two loops around a pair of soccer fields, with a little extra at the start and finish, for 1.5 miles. There are separate races for boys and girls. The boys will run first in a field of close to 100 runners from the three schools.

A GROUNDBREAKING RUNNING PROGRAM

This race marks another new running experience for Danny as he breaks ground, week by week, month by month, for autistic children, thought to be incapable of rigorous exercise and almost unheard of in a sport like cross-country or track and field. From his running start in fourth- and fifth-grade PE class with Mantone taking him by the hand, Danny progressed to weekend runs of 4 miles on a track supervised by his mom, 5-milers around a nature preserve with Mantone, summer 5K races with Mantone literally holding on to him, sixth-grade track on his own around a 400-meter oval, and now seventh-grade cross-country. In the process, Danny has been smashing commonly accepted boundaries in what doctors call the fastest-growing developmental disability in the United States. According to the Centers for Disease Control, 1 in every 152 American kids has some form of autism (in New Jersey it's 1 in 94), and 1.5 million youngsters suffer from the disease. Boys, perhaps because of testosterone, represent a higher percentage of autistic children, according to doctors.

Autism is a brain disorder encompassing a broad range of language, learning, and behavioral issues on a spectrum of severity. The epidemic has become front-page news and about every other week or so fills "the hour" with *Larry King*. Most treatment involves behavioral and language therapy with emphasis on early intervention; in some cases, special diets and nutritional supplements are advised. The cause is unknown amid heated argument over what it might be.

Unfortunately, the national debate and its political fury seem to have obscured efforts to enhance the lives of autistic youngsters with mainstream activities. Recognizing that autistic children benefit from seeing how other children act, some schools have begun more mainstreaming of special-needs youngsters. Elsewhere in New Jersey, for example, in the Fair Lawn district, autistic children at age 3 enter a Stepping-Stones program to prepare them for the possibility of mainstreaming as they get older.

Diagnosed with autism at 4, Danny entered a self-contained autistic class in kindergarten in Marlboro and has continued with that setup through the elementary grades and into middle school. He has taken "adaptive" PE classes with autistic classmates. While Danny has not been mainstreamed in the classroom, he was ushered in that direction by Mantone, who saw his physical ability and desire to run, which ultimately led him to the middle school track and cross-country teams—mainstreaming at its best.

"Running seems to have a calming effect on Danny," Anne Marie tells me as race time looms on the cross-country course. "I also notice more language. He seems to have a higher level of understanding. The other day I told him that he had track practice. He corrected me and said, 'No, it's cross-country.' That's a fine distinction."

OPPORTUNITIES FOR AUTISTIC KIDS

Special-needs kids have been involved in sports for years, ever since the Kennedys got the Special Olympics off the ground in the 1960s. But it has not been until recently, as differentness has more easily come out of the closet, that these youngsters have begun participating on regular varsity sports teams. Perhaps the best known—at least after his appearance on *Larry King Live*—is J. J. MacElwain, a high-functioning autistic boy who played high school basketball in upstate New York, sank a winning basket in a big game, and wrote a book about it.

In running, Danny is setting the pace in an exciting new development that offers great hope for the autistic community. Others are taking up the call. In a visit to Lynbrook Elementary School in Springfield, Virginia (see chapter 4), I met another autistic athlete, Chuck, a fifth grader, who'd completed the Marine Corps Marathon Healthy Kids Fun Run in Washington, D.C., in October 2007, along with 171 of his classmates. As with Danny, it took enterprising and persistent adults to get Chuck moving into the mainstream. Kathy Ray, the school's speech and language pathologist who'd worked with Chuck since kindergarten, convinced the boy's parents, who were reluctant at first. Ray clinched the deal when she told Chuck she'd run the mile with him. He agreed, and his parents did too.

However, Marine officials were not sure about having an adult in their kids-only event. The Lynbrook PE teacher who'd spearheaded the school's running program, Richard Dexter, was able to get the Marines on board. Dexter's father was a lifelong military man who'd worked at the Pentagon, and Richard, a former army brat, spoke the Marines' language.

Kathy and Chuck submitted their race applications together. It was the first race for both. Ray was hardly a runner, but she understood what running could do for Chuck. "He wanted to be like the other kids," said Ray. "He wanted to do what they were doing." I saw that myself when I visited Lynbook and watched Chuck copy his classmates' jumping jacks in a regular PE class.

So Kathy and Chuck ran the mile in the pack of kids. Kathy held a water bottle for Chuck. When Chuck felt winded, he walked. When he ran, the Marines cheered him and he picked up his pace. At the finish, Chuck got a medal and a goody bag. There were hugs and tears all around. Best of all, Chuck could attend the big pizza party the school principal had promised the participants. Chuck, said Ray, was thrilled to be in the group.

Since then, said Ray, "Chuck has been more willing to try new things and shown a heightened sense of self-worth." And the two of them were planning to run the Healthy Kids Fun Run again in October 2008.

"This is all new to me," says Sue Webster before taking a strategic position on the cross-country trail to make sure Danny doesn't veer off course. She tells me that in her nine years teaching at a highly regarded school for autistic youngsters in Princeton, running was never brought up.

Webster has seen dramatic changes in Danny that she attributes to his running. "If you see him running, there's no difference whatsoever between him and his peers," she says with wonder. "I've never seen him so focused."

Just as every child is different, every autistic child is different, and preconceived notions often hold these special children back. When I spoke with Danny's physician, Dr. Susan Levy of the Children's Hospital of Philadelphia, she told me that it had never occurred to her to suggest running; after all, she'd never heard of an autistic child who ran. Dr. Levy, who heads the hospital's Regional Autism Center, characterized Danny as somewhat above average in autistic functioning. When Anne Marie told her of Danny's running, Dr. Levy gave her blessing with no reservations. "It was thrilling," she said. In her office, she has a picture of Danny in his track uniform (see interview, page 221).

Danny has qualities that help him in his running, like good muscle tone and physical dexterity, as well as qualities that running brings out in him, like an outgoing personality. "Danny seems to attract people. Everybody likes him," says his father, Eric.

Running has opened a new world for Danny. If he had been left to his own devices in fourth grade without the influence of a visionary like Pat Mantone, he would not be shaking people's hands, giving high fives, training like a varsity athlete, and poised to run a 1.5-mile cross-country race on his own with a big crowd cheering him on.

AUTISM ISSUES AFFECT RACE START

The start of a race is a problem for Danny. Whether it's the crack of a gun or a whistle that will send the field off, Danny has a delay in processing the sound, allowing the other runners, in effect, a head start. Also, because he's a visual learner, he tends to watch the other youngsters as a signal to get going. There's also a fear factor in the loud noise of a gun. In addition, Danny has the common autistic tendency to stay on the periphery of a crowd, avoiding physical closeness. Keeping Danny on the side may actually serve as a safety measure in a big cross-country or road race field; if he was positioned in the middle, his delay could cause him to be knocked over by runners from behind.

Team Danny covers all bases. When Sinisi practices a whistle start with Danny running by himself, she finds he does better. When Mantone runs with Danny in 5K road races, she introduces him to other runners on the starting line so he'll feel more at ease in the crowd. At cross-country meets, Mantone, who knows many of the team members, will pick out a child to stand behind Danny "and give him a little nudge when the gun goes off." She says, "Kids love to help."

The race official steadies the field for the start. The whistle shrieks and the boys take off. Danny, wearing number 21, gets no push-off today. He loses a few seconds and moves into a steady pace while many others, possessed by the impulse of youth, fly out fast. The coaching mantra of "even pace" is perfect for Danny. Sue runs to the top of a small hill for a broad view of the field. Danny's the only boy with a headband.

Marlboro dominates the race. A little guy from the team motors along in the lead at a brisk pace. After the first loop, Danny runs by, about a minute behind the leader, to whooping cheers.

"Fantastic," calls Sue.

"My son won't stop. Look at him," shouts Anne Marie.

"When he took off he was smiling. He's come so far it's unbelievable," says his aunt Kathy.

"When he gets his next neuro check," says Anne Marie, "I can't wait for the doctor to get a look at him."

On the second loop, Danny picks up his pace, passing other runners. At one point he veers in the wrong direction but is led back. He rallies with the finish in view and crosses the line in thirty-fifth place in the field of ninety-three boys. Danny's time is 13:20, fully four minutes ahead of the slowest kids. He looks tired but not breathless.

"Look at his race," says Pat. "He ran the second half faster than the first."

Danny's friend Nick, who finished thirty-first and helped keep track of Danny, gives him a high five, telling him, "You ran very fast."

Initially, not all of the Marlboro squad was that keen on Danny. Middle school can be brutal. "If you wear your hair wrong one day," says Sinisi, "you are the butt of everyone's jokes." When Danny joined the track team in sixth grade, Sinisi did not want to draw attention to him and said nothing. But after noticing some under-the-breath ridicule, she gathered the team for a lecture, saying, "I bet Dan could find a couple of things that you do that's funny."

RUNNING FAST, MAKING FRIENDS

Soon, says Sinisi, when the kids saw Danny's running prowess, "he was everybody's best friend." The team has warmed to Danny's quirky moments, like when he gets in someone's face with the refrain, "I keep running." Sinisi says that as hard as it is to teach tolerance to this age group, the other kids now accept Danny as a peer. "I get goose bumps just thinking about it," she says.

This is not a time for hesitancy. It's not a time to wait for a consensus on autism's cause. It's not a time to question what an autistic child can accomplish. Let's not lose a generation of kids. Let's get them moving: walking, running, and, yes, even racing. We just might find that this evolving, amorphous categorization need not hold these youngsters back—that the power of running can help them gain language, learning ability, and social skills to become, at their best, almost as "typical" as anyone. We just might find that running is a perfect antidote for children slowed by an ill-defined strangeness at an early age.

Danny was born on January 31, 1995. He weighed 8 pounds 11 ounces and, says Anne Marie, "was perfect." Her pregnancy was normal except for one thing: a 24-week ultrasound showed bilateral cysts (bubbles) on Danny's brain. Further tests indicated everything was fine and that the cysts had dissolved. "It's interesting," says Anne Marie, an attorney and partner in a New Jersey law firm, "that a boy in Danny's autistic class who happens to be his best friend had the same condition."

Between ages 2 and 3, Danny, an only child, seemed to ignore other children in his midst and have more tantrums than other kids, and while he was able to say words and identify letters and numbers he was not forming sentences. Since Anne Marie and her husband, Eric, a chiropractor, had no other children to compare him to, they were not yet alarmed, especially since doctors held off with an autism assessment. Then one day at nursery school Danny walked on, instead of around, a napping child.

At 4, Danny was declared autistic by a New Jersey physician, who sent the family to Children's Hospital of Philadelphia, noted for its autism care. Later, Eric would blame the vaccines Danny received. But Anne Marie maintains that even before getting the MMR vaccine Danny did not have a "functional point" with his hand, a key autism indicator.

"We were devastated," says Anne Marie.

Eric felt the loss of father-and-son activity, saying, "Things I expected to do with Danny would not come to be."

Checking the state Education Department Web site, they learned that Marlboro, one town over from where they were living, had one of the highest special education budgets of any district. They moved, Danny started kindergarten, and four years and two schools later, Danny entered Marlboro Elementary. The principal, Jon Shutman, took Danny by the hand and walked him around the school so he would know what to expect. "The man is a god," Anne Marie says.

ONE TEACHER'S PERSONAL APPROACH

If the principal is a god, then Pat Mantone must be a goddess. To a large extent, autism problems lie not with the child but with unyielding adult attitudes. Foot soldiers in the war against old ideas, like Mantone, can make all the difference. In her thirty-one years at Marlboro El, Mantone, 55, has collected a slew of teaching awards, and banners in the gym attest to the school's eight state championship titles in the Presidential Physical Fitness Challenge. Those titles have come despite the district's meager 40 minutes of PE once every six days—only thirty periods per school year.

With a pressure-free teaching style, Mantone incorporates running into every activity in a jam-packed period. "I have to get kids to love it," she says. Like she loves it: a runner since college with thirty marathons to her credit, Mantone trains close to 10 miles a day, most of it at 5:30 in the morning before school. She enters the building boosted, she says, by "a runner's high."

From his start with Mantone in fourth grade, Danny caught the vibe. Mantone started the autistic children walking in place. She had to pick up their legs at first, then they did it on their own. She added jumping and had them move through hula hoops for locomotive skills. "Danny's ability," says Mantone, "was that whatever I set up he could keep going." Sitting on a big ball, Danny could bounce up and down repeatedly, showing leg strength, balance, and coordination. While moving, Danny would talk to Tigger, a character in a Winnie the Pooh video.

Autistic students in New Jersey receive 40 minutes a day of adaptive PE. Parents learn they can never take anything for granted. Early in seventh-grade track, Danny was sent home from practice one day because there was no special-education aide for him. Based on the resolution of an earlier dispute, an aide was required to be funded for all team practices. Anne Marie complained to a special services supervisor and within days an aide was present.

Dr. Levy said Anne Marie is a dynamo who "has done phenomenal things with Danny." Anne Marie has learned about running (promising to start herself) and can speak about "junk" miles, a coach's term for added workouts that are unnecessary and may cause injury. Danny's only injury so far has come from his first pair of trail shoes, which bruised his Achilles tendon. After switching to other models, he has been pain-free.

For her part, Mantone has had no formal training in autism. "I experimented," she says. Everything she did had to be demonstrated because the kids could not understand if she said, "Jump." She had to physically handle them. "That's how they learn. I was exhausted. Some of these kids weighed more than me."

Finally, she got the kids running, in the gym and outside on the field. She pushed the children from behind to keep them moving. She did not have to push Danny. "He chose to run," says Mantone. "We would run around the playground together and I would stop at something and ask him what color it was. We would see a house and I would ask him about his house. He became more verbal." When the class did a scavenger hunt, Danny led the way, racing to the pine cones. "I think Danny is a kinesthetic learner. He needs to smell it, touch it, taste it."

No wonder Danny loves running. It involves all the senses.

"There's no reason why just about any autistic youngster can't run," says Mantone. "But they're not going to get up and start it on their own."

DANNY'S GIFT INSPIRES OTHERS

Danny's spring track coach at Marlboro Middle, Glenn Odato, like Sinisi a special-ed teacher, says that in more than twenty years at the school he's never seen an autistic youngster like Danny. In the adaptive PE class, when Odato first had the kids work with a soccer ball, Danny wouldn't stop running. "I saw he loved it. His heels were coming up nicely. He has a gift to run," he says.

Odato told Danny's father about his son's athletic ability, and one day Eric stopped by school to observe a PE class. "Glenn gave Danny a basketball," Eric says. "He missed the first two shots but then every one went in."

Danny's already become a role model for another autistic child who needs more prompting to run. His classmate Bryan has started joining him for laps of the high school track. First Bryan walked, then he ran, then he joined the school track squad. "He comes to practice," says Sinisi. "Maybe he can eventually excel like Danny." Anne Marie is lobbying parents of other kids in the class to join in. Imagine someday an entire class of autistic children running.

The school teams could not have a stronger advocate than Anne Marie, who considers track and cross-country "the most important therapy of all." She says, "Track kids are not like other athletes. They don't compete against one another but against themselves. Where else could I find typical children to interact with Danny and treat him like a peer?"

Anne Marie tells me that if time issues developed and something had to be cut, she would sooner cut Danny's speech therapy or behavior therapy than his running. She says that Danny's local pediatrician was awed by his progress in his latest exam. "He was perfectly behaved. He used his language and was focused and attentive. The doctor was amazed," she says.

THE BEST THERAPY OF ALL

It is clear from watching Danny on the cross-country course, around the track, in summer road races, or training on a nature trail that every mile covered is a mile to behold, that this is a boy entering adolescence who is proud of himself and regarded by teammates not as an oddity but as a runner, an athlete, and a good one. His teacher, Sue Webster, says, "What sets him apart from other autistic athletes I've worked with and seen is that he loves what he does. He is not being forced to run or pushed in any way."

As challenging as the team environment can be for Danny— the complexities of "social negotiation," as Dr. Levy put it, in a large group of excitable teens—the team offers Danny a certain security, as the running routines are pleasingly familiar to him. The classroom and school corridors are even more of a litmus test of Danny's progress.

When other students see Danny in the hallways they call his name and give him high fives. Danny responds by saying their name or asking them their name. "I hear my son is a celebrity in school," says Anne Marie. She notes that one time in a restaurant the school soccer coach pointed out to other diners with pride: "That's Danny!"

Early in sixth grade, in late fall, Anne Marie was called into school to meet with the child study team and review Danny's Individualized Education Plan (IEP). All his academic and social goals for the year had been met. New, higher goals could be set. "I believe that was because of his running and what it did for him," says Mantone. "It woke Danny up."

DANNY'S PERFORMANCE BREAKTHROUGHS

As if training for the Olympics, Danny won't miss a workout. On a family trip to the Caribbean, Danny runs 4 miles a day on a treadmill in the hotel fitness center (and at home is up to 7.2 mph, 8:25 per mile, at a 1 percent incline, for six miles). At practice, he doesn't want to stop, approaching the coach and asking, "Mrs. Sinisi, I do more running?" Sue Webster says she can hear Danny coaching himself while running. "He repeats quietly, 'Keep on running, keep on running.'"

His second favorite sport is rock climbing.

Danny has a better work ethic than half the team—and now some faster times. When he started track in sixth grade, he ran a mile time trial in 11 minutes and got his race times down to 9 minutes. In seventh-grade track, he ran a preseason time trial in 7:30. Sinisi says that by the end of middle school, in eighth grade, Danny could be running under 7 minutes for the mile. "When his peers ask him how he runs in track," says Webster, "his response is, 'I run fast.'" In eighth-grade cross-country, he improved to 10:36 for 1.5 miles.

Another breakthrough for an autistic child: Danny is not just participating but achieving high performance. Mantone recently gave Anne Marie a plyometrics plan for Danny to follow. These are advanced exercises likes hopping, jumping for height, and "butt kicks" done by top-flight athletes seeking total fitness. Anne Marie has already notified the high school that Danny will be coming out for the varsity team. And the school, Howell High, which has the district's high school autism center, has an excellent squad.

It's hard to believe that all this started tentatively with Pat and Danny linking arms on the playground. Pat has been holding Danny's hand, at least figuratively, ever since. At his IEP meeting prior to leaving Marlboro El for middle school, Pat went out on a limb and told the assemblage—school psychologist, learning disability consultant, and Danny's parents—that Danny was a good runner and should go out for the middle school team.

"I almost fell off my chair," reports Anne Marie. "I said, 'Excuse me? Run? But . . . Danny has autism.'" Pat described how she and Danny had been running together in PE and how being part of a school team would help him with social skills. It was agreed, but the case manager insisted that Danny skip fall cross-country to get adjusted to middle school, and go out for track the following spring.

SPECIAL NURTURING OF SPECIAL NEEDS

With forward-thinking adults behind him or her, any special-needs child can go the extra mile. John Fisher, an autistic boy in Elmhurst, Illinois, who is higher-functioning than Danny, found the same transforming experience at York High School, where the boys' track and cross-country coach, Joe Newton, nurtured him for four years. Fisher did not speak as a child and was given a diagnosis of pervasive developmental disorder (PDD), a mild form of autism. A psychologist told John's parents that "the best we could hope for is that he's going to push a broom." After intensive therapy John began speaking, and after running at York, known for its national rankings, John could stand in front of a packed auditorium, microphone in hand, and deliver a team valedictory following a championship meet. John graduated in 2006 and went on to a nearby junior college, DuPage, where he has been a five-time all-American in track and cross-country and is studying applied fire sciences to become a firefighter.

In Duxbury, Vermont, a Down syndrome girl, Gracie Kirpan, competes on the Harwood Union track and cross-country squads. A runner since seventh grade and one of eleven children, ten of whom were adopted (including Gracie), she was born with a hole in her heart and is practically deaf. The Harwood coach, John Kerrigan, said he treats Gracie like everyone else on his team, which she prefers. If the team runs an 11-mile loop, so does Gracie; it just takes her longer and she does some walking. Accompanied by a special-education aide, she does the loop backward, so other runners will pick her up and also keep their eyes on her. "Cross-country running," said Harwood principal Sue Duprat, "is one of the very few programs at any school that can accommodate such a vast range of student abilities and needs."

In March 2008 I spoke with a legally blind runner, Markeith Price of Baltimore, at the Nike Indoor Nationals high school championships in Landover, Maryland. Price, then a senior at Mt. St. Joseph High School, competed in the 400 meters despite having optic atrophy in both eyes since birth. (This is the same eye condition that afflicts New York governor David A. Patterson, himself a runner.) Price said that the nerves in his eyes that connect to the brain were not fully developed. "I've learned to deal with it," he said. "I haven't made it a hindrance."

Price, who started running as a young child, hoped to compete in the 2008 Paralympics in Beijing, China, the worldwide event for disabled athletes that follows the Olympic Games. In 2007, Price competed in three events in a regional Paralympics event in São Paulo, Brazil. He was planning on running in college and studying fashion. Price showed some style in Landover, competing in multicolored calf-length stockings as opposed to drab athletic sweat socks.

"HIP, HIP, HOORAY" ON THE TRACK

Danny would appreciate those socks. He's got that cool signature headband, a retro look, and his own sense of style. The headband—this time white—was on display in mid-2007 at Monmouth Battleground Park in Manalapan when Danny participated in the Freehold Area Running Club's summer racing series. The club has an array of kids' events up to a mile (see chapter 3), but Pat felt Danny was fit enough to run the adult 5K, even in the 90°-plus temperatures. With sixth-grade track over and fall cross-country coming, Pat had given Anne Marie a summer training program for Danny. She took him to the high school track four evenings a week. He would run 16 laps, four miles, without stopping.

To get him started, Pat ran with him at the track. "He would be laughing and saying 'Hip, hip, hooray,'" Pat recalls. "It was a fight to take him off the track." She nurtured Danny's desire for distance with weekend jaunts around the 5-mile nature trail at the Manasquan Reservoir as Anne Marie rode a bike behind them with a water bottle. "I'd point out things, like deer, horses," says Pat, who held Danny's hand on the sandy path. "When Danny would say 'horses' to me, I knew he wanted to run the reservoir route." Danny got his times down to 50 minutes.

That approach translated into the weekly summer evening races. Pat would run with Danny holding his hand, pushing him up a hill, a buffer in the crowded field. In the heat, this was Danny's toughest challenge yet. "When Danny's pace would slow, I would reach out with my hand and he would grab it," says Pat. "Like other autistic children, Danny takes everything literally. If I told him to 'push harder,' he would squeeze my hand harder. I learned to say 'faster.' I have also learned to interpret Danny's facial and body language. We can have an entire conversation without any words spoken."

Without letup, and even picking up his pace after seeing the

3-mile sign, Danny charged across the finish, with Pat on his right shoulder. His time for the first race was 30:53. Then he ran 33:12 (a 100°, humid day), 28:59, 28:53, 29:06, and 27:10, his best (further improved to 26:01, 8:20 per mile, in the next summer series).

By the fall in seventh-grade cross-country, many of Danny's self-stimulating autistic behaviors had almost been eliminated. The once-prevalent hand-flapping, self-talk, OCD-like repetition, eye contact avoidance, and crowd fears had lessened. "Running has taken Danny out of his shell," concludes Webster.

His favorite workouts, said Sinisi, are what she calls "long and lovely days": distance runs of up to 40 minutes at a relaxed, conversational pace. With Danny's help, the Marlboro boys' team won its first league trophy, placing third in the nine-team division.

Preparing Danny for school track, Mantone practiced running laps with him. "You have to practice something over and over with an autistic youngster. They need to build those neuro pathways into the brain," she says. That includes all phases of running: stretching, uniform, water bottle, running partners, forming a template that the child can draw upon. "They thrive on the routines," she says. "Throw them a curve ball and you'll have a problem."

TWO WORLDS, DIFFERENT FOCUS

Danny gets a curve ball in his first seventh-grade track meet in April 2008. Competing in the 1,600 meters, he musters little focus, jogs instead of racing, almost stops at different points, gets lapped, and finishes with a 9-minute time—a much slower pace than he's run in longer races. He's cheered by the crowd and smiling afterward, so who can be disappointed? It seems that the four laps throw him off. Unlike cross-country trails with spectators along the way to scoot him on and other runners near him at all times, he gets mentally lost on the track after the small field takes off and he is basically alone. "He needs constant attention to keep running hard," says Pat. "Autistic children live in their own world, and it is our job to bring them out."

Seemingly small details can count for a lot. Pat tells me that Danny used to refer to himself in the third person, saying things like "It's Danny's turn," indicative of existing in his own, separate world. "The biggest thing I've been noticing," she says, "is that he's becoming his own person. Recently he told his mom, 'I run fast too. I run.' That's a big breakthrough, referring to himself that way. Now he's got himself in *our* world."

Sinisi also struggles for insights into Danny's behavior. But in cross-country she has a hundred teens to supervise. At one practice, Sinisi gets nervous when she notices Danny wheezing during a run. She questions him but then realizes, "Oh my gosh, he can't tell me what's wrong." She calls Anne Marie for help. Another day, Danny keeps telling her, "More knees, more knees," and lifting his knees. Sinisi wonders: *Does his knee hurt?* Eventually, she understands that Danny wants to do more knee exercises, like the skipping drills Sinisi instructed. "My slogan with Dan," she says, "is that no matter how much you think you're going to teach someone, they're going to teach you."

When Danny runs with Pat, it's hard to say who the teacher is. "Being with Danny gives me so much," she says. "I'm constantly learning from him. When I ran the whole summer with him I was probably my happiest."

Pat looks forward to the day, perhaps coming soon, when she will no longer be able to keep up with Danny, when he will need to take *her* by the hand and lead her. Pat knows she'll have to stay in good shape because she and Danny have set a long-term goal: running the New York City Marathon together when he turns 18.

Autistic Children and Running:
A Medical Viewpoint

Interview with Danny's physician, Susan E. Levy, founder and director of the Regional Autism Center at the Children's Hospital of Philadelphia (CHOP). Dr. Levy is a developmental pediatrician specializing in neurodevelopmental disabilities.

Q. With statistics showing 1 in 150 children diagnosed with autism, is the disease an epidemic?
A. Children's Hospital was one of thirteen autism centers contributing to that finding, which came out in February 2007. Autism is more common than it used to be, but it is not an epidemic. Since autism was first described fifty years ago, the criteria for diagnoses have changed, and each year the description has broadened. Originally the criteria were narrow. Now many people are looking at it differently, as more of a category of disabilities of social and communicative disorders.

Q. What were your expectations when you first saw Danny at age 5?
A. The goal was to make him as functional as possible. I did not think he would be able to participate in a sport like running, especially on a team. That's hard, complex. You have social negotiation, listening to people. I was pleasantly surprised when I heard about it.

(continued)

Q. Early on, you had no impression of Danny as a potential athlete?
A. No.

Q. Other than Danny, have you ever seen another autistic youngster in a running program?
A. No. I have had kids who are great musicians, have perfect pitch, and can sing and play. I have had some athletes, but not like Danny.

Q. Many autistic children have weak muscles, or hypotonia.
A. Yes, a fair amount have low muscle tone, what we used to call "double-jointed." Not everyone with low muscle tone has poor coordination. But even among kids who are higher-functioning, problems with coordination are fairly common. Danny is unusual. It's cool.

Q. Did you have any medical concerns when you learned of Danny's running?
A. None. Autism is not a physical disability. With a Down syndrome child, you have the potential for some physical problems like spine instability. Autism doesn't carry the same kind of issues. The issues that might come up with autism are a matter of supervision. I don't know that I'd feel comfortable with Danny running far distances on his own.

Q. Danny's running seems to be having a profound effect on him.
A. It's like his social skills training. We advise families to find something that the child is good at, where they can be with peers and learn how to deal with people. An individual-and-team sport like running is wonder-

ful and so healthy. Running is a repetitive activity. And I'm sure that on some level Danny gets his endorphins going. He feels good. Those things are good for kids with autism.

Q. Why are repetition and routine so important to autistic children?
A. I don't know that anybody knows why. It is one of the core characteristics that autistic children engage in repetitive behavior. Whether it's part of being obsessive-compulsive, or ritualistic, feeling more comfortable when they know what's going to happen next.

Q. Danny's inspiration, Pat Mantone, is not an autism expert but learned by having a passionate interest in Danny. Is that a good sign that you don't need experts but caring people?
A. I'm encouraged by it, but I don't think it happens that commonly. Danny doesn't have a lot of behavior problems. He has been managed superbly by his parents. He's more malleable. Some other kids we follow have more significant behavior issues—attention, focus, aggression. I think it was brilliant that Pat picked up on something Danny would like.

Q. What brain malfunction occurs in autism?
A. There are a number of theories. One is that some areas that connect different parts of the brain don't work as well. It's not clear.

Q. But this does not always occur at birth.
A. About one-third of children with autism have symptoms right from birth. About one-third have gradual

(continued)

onset. About one-third appear to be fine, then somewhere between 18 months to 2 years, they lose either language and/or social skills. We think it's predetermined.

Q. Since Danny has improved in various areas of functioning, is something "good" happening to his brain?
A. It would seem so. The only way we know is, how it's working when we see him. At CHOP, we are expanding our research and are doing some special imaging studies and functional MRI studies of how the brain is working. Over the next five years we'll get a better sense of how the brain is working in children with autism.

Q. What have you noticed in Danny?
A. I see him every six to twelve months, and so have seen him a few times since his running began. When I'm tracking his progress, a lot of that is what his mom tells me about school. I have seen a positive trend in his visits. He seems a little more "connected." In earlier years, when I first saw him, he was a little disconnected. Now he's more responsive, tuning into people in his environment; earlier, he was more distant and self-involved.

Q. Is running the main reason for Danny's improvement?
A. I would think so. I don't know if it's just the running per se. Because of the running, people are treating him typically [that is, like everyone else] and are excited about him, and he's getting positive feedback and positive attention. With his running, people look at him as a more successful person. So people treat him differently.

Q. How others treat you is critical?

A. He's treated equally by peers. He feels good about himself. He looks healthy. He feels healthy. All of those factors . . . I think a lot of it is how people view him. And if you think he's doing great, then you might push him more.

Q. Can Danny sense negative treatment?

A. He senses it. Just because he has autism doesn't mean he's not tuned in to how people are treating him, or different emotions.

Q. You mentioned endorphins. Can Danny intellectually appreciate the good feelings of running?

A. I don't know. You have to judge it indirectly. Is he smiling? Is he happier? Does he seem more peaceful? Look at the secondary effects. I don't think that cognitively he understands that "running is really good for me."

Q. Danny has made vast improvement in a short time. What next?

A. I expect him to continue to improve.

Q. Couldn't the majority of autistic youngsters benefit from running?

A. It depends on their cognitive skills and where their associated problems are. Sensory issues are very common with kids with autism. Some are insurmountable. We encourage all our families to get their children involved in sports, physical activities, especially when

(continued)

they're younger. Swimming is another good individual-and-team sport. There are sets of rules, routines, and if the autistic kids know what the rules are, it's so much easier for them to interact with peers.

Q. I was surprised to find out that Danny had been involved in a swim program. Isn't swimming complex?
A. Swimming has a rhythmic nature, and kids love the water. There are rules, routines: swim up and back. In a relay, you take turns. It's similar to running.

Q. Is there any reason why a good many parents of autistic children should not experiment with running?
A. I think it might be helpful. Danny is a good example for autistic families.

▶ Groovin' with Danny on a Sunday Afternoon

On a lovely early spring day for running—50°, light breeze, plenty of sun—Danny, Pat Mantone, and I meet at the 5-mile Perimeter Trail of Manasquan Reservoir, a recreation area and wildlife sanctuary in a nearby town. Danny, who recently turned 13, is wearing his signature headband to keep sweat away from his eyes. Before running, Pat takes Danny through a dozen stretching exercises: some sitting, some standing, working all the muscles. Pat demonstrates, sometimes positioning Danny's arms or legs, and he follows to the letter. Each exercise is held to a count of 20. Danny calls off the numbers with each stretch. Danny even does forward and backward jumps, feet together, with no assistance needed.

Despite running 4 miles the day before on a track and just

getting over the flu a few days ago, Danny is ready to run the path, made of cinder and gravel and filled with mountain bikers and dog walkers. Pat runs the path most mornings, covering two loops, or 10 miles. Danny's mom, Anne Marie, had told me that when Danny was running the path some months ago he got his times down from over an hour to 50 minutes.

Pat walks Danny across the parking lot to the trailhead. She doesn't want to "teach" Danny that it's okay to run in a parking lot. She anticipates everything. "You have to," she says.

I expect a 10-minute-mile pace, but Danny darts out briskly, head high, knees up, arms close to his side. "He's so different from when we first started," says Pat. "I would be holding his hand. Now he likes to run by himself." That independence is a breakthrough.

Our trio settles into a groove: Danny on the left, Pat in the middle, me on the right. We pass a dog walker. "See the dog? What color is the dog?" Pat calls to Danny. He repeats: "See the dog, see the dog . . ." Pat says, "Only one time," and he stops.

The first of many short hills arrives. "Lean into the hill, Danny, lean in," says Pat.

Danny's smiling. At times, he picks up his pace spontaneously. When he does, his smile widens.

Now the downhill. "Fast," says Pat. "Open up. Good boy."

The pace feels like 8 minutes and change per mile. "Running on a treadmill has helped him," says Pat, referring to his recent running on vacation in Jamaica. "It forces him to run at a certain pace."

When the sun is hidden, a chill gathers and Danny pulls his sleeves over his hands. One runner trots by shirtless. We are all wishing for summer. Pat says that the thinner, dryer winter air was not good for Danny's asthma.

The first mile is 8:37. "Looking good, Daniel."

The path narrows near 2 miles and Pat must pull Danny into single file behind her so he won't run into bicyclists. She refers to his difficulty with spatial awareness. A cold crosswind smacks us. Danny's knee lift remains high, a sign of energy in reserve.

The 2-mile split is 17:40, 9:03 for the second mile. "Look at the horse," calls Pat. Danny does his repeat routine. A minute later, when Danny sags, Pat grabs his hand for the first time. "Are you tired?" she asks. "Yes," he says, but it's hard to know. A few seconds later, she says, "Feeling better?" Dan says yes. She lets go. Maybe he just wanted a hand to hold.

Danny's cheeks turn crimson. We're halfway home. The sun returns and Danny tires. Pat stops and removes his sweatshirt, tying it around her waist.

"Feeling better?"

"Yes."

We curve out of the woods and into an open stretch, getting a broad view of the reservoir. Bare branches jut out of the water. "This is my favorite part in the morning," Pat says. "The sun comes up right here."

Then we're back in the woods with the next hill waiting. "Pump, Danny, pump."

Few kids on Danny's middle school team could run 5 miles like this. I tell Pat that everything she's doing with Danny is cutting-edge. "We're learning as we go," Pat says.

Danny hits 3 miles in 27:06. He opens up again on a downhill. I suggest to Pat that Danny is not able to assess fatigue and really know the level of strain in his running. She agrees. That would mean that as Danny gains more exertion awareness he'll run even better. "He's learning that now," says Pat. "C'mon, buddy."

Suddenly, Danny sprints *up* a hill, dodging what a horse left behind, and continues the pace on the descent. "Blow out," Pat orders. She means for Danny to breath hard through his nose. While running he doesn't spit or do the runner's finger-nostril nose blow, and Pat doesn't want to teach him that for fear he'll do it in public.

Heading toward 4 miles. "Keep it up," says Pat. "You're going to run your personal best today."

The sun's warmth is comforting but Danny labors a bit, grabbing his fingers at chest level. His eyes show distress. Pat runs a few yards ahead to lead him. I'm at his side. He stops for a breather. Pat grabs his hand. He's okay with that. With her left hand on Danny's back, she helps push him up a hill.

The 4-mile time is 36:27. "This is uncharted territory," says Pat—an autistic child with a year and a half worth of formal running experience doing a 5-mile run at a pace most adults could not match.

The last hill comes and Danny flies down. "Wooooo!" shrieks Pat.

The trail flattens out and the finish looms. Pat urges Danny on. He can tell he's almost home. "Soon we're going to see Mommy," Pat says.

Danny perks up, returning to his initial, knee-lifting gait.

"Are you having fun?" Pat says in a valedictory.

"Yes."

Danny hits the finish in 46:32, his best time by over three minutes. We greet Mom and get a drink.

"Don't you get energy from running with him?" Pat says to me.

"Did you see how much Danny appreciates running?" Anne Marie says to me.

Yes.

11

Running with All Sports

In the off-season, we have a program in which we alternate sprints and jumping rope one day with running a mile and a half on the track plus stadium steps another day.

—LISA ARCE, GIRLS' VOLLEYBALL COACH OF 2007 NATIONAL
CHAMPION MIRA COSTA HIGH IN CALIFORNIA

Ken Potter, the football coach at Oregon state champion Jesuit High in Portland, gives his team a 3-mile time trial at the start of the season in late August to make sure the Crusaders are in shape for the fall campaign. "Endurance is important in football," says Potter. "The whole team knows we have the 3-miler and they have to be ready for it by running over the summer." Debbie Schwartz, girls' softball coach at state-ranked Toms River East High in New Jersey, gives her players a six-week program of sprints and distance, working up to a 2-mile run while advising younger athletes to play running games, to avoid injuries like pulled muscles. Lisa Arce, girls' volleyball coach at California's Mira Costa High, ranked number one in the country in 2007, has her team alternate days of sprinting with days of 2-mile runs during the fall season. She says that younger players should do the same, limiting distance to 5-minute runs, or a little more than a half mile, for less impact.

Whether you play in recreational leagues or on travel teams, try out for middle school or high school teams, attend specialized camps, work with personal trainers, or just choose up sides with friends, running ability is crucial in all sports. Running builds the body—conditioning the legs, heart, lungs, virtually all muscle groups—to move on a court, field, or other venue and have the stamina to handle practices and games and throughout the whole season. Running also enables you to avoid fatigue that compromises hard-won skills while gaining the strength to minimize injury. "Conditioned athletes suffer less injury, and less severe injuries, and recover faster," says Evan Pickman, a former college coach and longtime NBA scout with the Los Angeles Clippers who lectures at youth basketball camps.

Whether the recommended fitness program emphasizes distance running, sprints, drills, or running games—like going foul pole to foul pole in baseball—the following award-winning coaches, and one college athlete, in fourteen sports provide expert advice to help you improve your game and reach your potential while having fun at the same time.

ALPINE SKIING: COACH STEVEN BERLACK

Credentials: Berlack is a coach in the junior program at Burke Academy in Vermont, a private high school combining alpine (downhill) ski racing instruction with an academic program.

Running commitment. Distance running is one of the best ways to build an aerobic base, which aids in recovery when skiing. In the course of a winter, the training load on a hill is huge. The body's ability to recover is largely based on its ability to transport oxygen, which is enhanced by running. For a youngster, the golden age of learning is between 7 and 13. Running at this age will build good habits for the future.

Distance running. A 12-year-old skier is on the hill for two and a half hours a day in training. To prepare for that, we recommend a six-month conditioning program starting in April, in which a 12-year-old, for example, will run 30 minutes a day three to five days a week at a relaxed, conversational pace. (To be "mountain strong," we also like kids hiking in the mountains, where steep, rocky terrain makes running difficult.)

Sprint work. Fast, repeated runs of 30, 60, and 90 seconds.

Competitive edge. There's no question that a modest but fit athlete can put a lot of competitors behind him in the last ten seconds of a run—which is all will and conditioning—just by holding his edge. A more "talented" athlete who lacks fitness will find his legs burning at the end.

Injury prevention. Knee pain is common in ski racing. Stronger skiers experience less fatigue, which can result in less risk to the knees.

Pushing the pace. Every spring in late May, we have the Green Mountain Run, a relay, from the Massachusetts border through Vermont to the Canadian border, 204 miles. Burke high school students run legs of 5 miles, and many youngsters also run with friends, doing as much as 30 miles in a twenty-four-hour period. To prepare for that, they train 3 to 7 miles, six days a week.

BASEBALL: COACH DON LANDOLPHI

Credentials: With forty years in coaching, Landolphi, who lives on Long Island, was assistant baseball coach of the 1995 U.S. Pan-American team, was assistant coach of the Italian national team for three years, and is a member of the American Baseball Coaches Hall of Fame.

Running commitment. Young players tend to run with choppy steps and need to learn how to stretch out their legs, running on the balls of their feet, to get down to first base and run the bases swiftly. At most positions, players need quickness more than aerobic endurance, with the main exception being the pitcher. Even though pitchers work only every fourth or fifth day, they use their legs as a foundation of strength. A teenage pitcher may throw 100 pitches or more in a game. A fit pitcher will experience less fatigue and, consequently, less arm strain.

Distance running. When I train older pitchers, I have them run from the left to right field foul poles and back, ten sets, which, at 100 yards per run, would amount to over a mile. This would be done a few days a week, on pitchers' off days. One pitcher whom I coached in Italy who is now with the Chicago Cubs would do a 30-minute run as a cool-down after working a game, to help reduce muscle fatigue.

Sprint work. To lengthen a choppy stride, practice running with a "leaping" stride from home plate to a point about 20 feet past first base. Be conscious of extending your legs. Also, run from home to first base twice, then to second base twice, then to third base twice, then finish with one hard run around the bases. Do these runs at about 95 percent of maximum effort. See if you can improve your time to first. The fastest major leaguers get from home to first in 4.2 seconds.

Competitive edge. Get game-ready by chasing fungos. With the player at home, the coach hits long balls to the outfield, and the player chases after them, then runs with the ball around the field, returning it to the coach. Repeat several times with brief rests between runs.

Injury prevention. With explosive running on the bases and quick bursts in the field, players' hamstring muscles take a beating. Conditioned athletes have less risk of hamstring problems.

Pushing the pace. Young players have a lot of fun doing relay races in which four kids are positioned at home and four are at second base and they race around the bases. This develops not only speed but also base-cutting skills.

BASKETBALL: COACH EVAN PICKMAN

Credentials: Pickman coached the College of Staten Island for twelve years, winning four City University titles, and since 1986 has been an NBA scout with the Los Angeles Clippers. He is a nationally known clinician and avid runner who has completed the New York City Marathon.

Running commitment. Basketball is a game of constant movement up and down the court, with forward, backward, and lateral running. Any youngster who wants to be in shape must develop cardiovascular endurance. With its stop-and-go action, basketball is more of an anaerobic than aerobic sport, and athletes must also acquire quickness and footwork with interval-style training. A quicker athlete can sometimes outplay an opponent who has more pure speed. Young players should combine two days of distance with two days of interval-style, stop-and-go drills per week.
Distance running. A young player, say 10 years old, should run 1 to 2 miles twice a week at a comfortable pace. High school players should do at least 3 miles every other day.
Sprint work. On nondistance days, the young athlete should do repeated baseline runs on the court. Run all-out baseline to baseline (84 feet for a regulation court) and back, trying to do it in under 15 seconds. Or run from one baseline to the other in 5 or 6 seconds, rest briefly, then run back. In the back-and-forth circuit, you also learn pivoting skills. Instead of making a "circular" turn or chopping your steps, reach with one foot, plant the foot, and push off with the planted foot while using the other foot in a lunging movement for the return.

Competitive edge. Run all-out from the baseline to the foul line and back; then from the baseline to midcourt and back; then from the baseline to the opposite foul line and back; then from the baseline to the opposite baseline and back. These are called "suicides" or "horses." Young players should do one circuit with older players doing two without stopping. Time them to see how you improve.

Injury prevention. Sprinting on the court without being in shape can result in a pulled muscle or torn Achilles tendon. Among girls, ACL injuries to the knee—anterior cruciate ligament—are prevalent because of girls' anatomy, how they land after jumping, and lack of strength (and strength imbalances) in the muscles supporting the knee.

Pushing the pace. For lateral quickness, stand in one corner of the baseline in a defensive stance (legs shoulder width apart, back straight, knees bent, one foot a little ahead, hands out, comfortable so you can "bounce") and, remaining in that stance, run in a sliding, sideways fashion to the foul line; then, facing the basket, plant your foot, pivot, and, keeping your stance, run in a sliding manner to midcourt. Be careful not to cross your legs or bring your feet together, a common fault of young players.

FIELD HOCKEY: COACH TISHA WERNER

Credentials: In 2006, Werner's Massapequa team won its first Long Island regional title and made the New York State Final Four and Werner was named Nassau County Coach of the Year by Newsday. In 2007, in her twelfth season, she earned her 100th victory.

Running commitment. The field measures 100 yards by 60 yards and there's not much subbing at the varsity level. Everyone must be fit, and the girls do a lot of running to get in shape for the fall season. One standard we want to see is the ability to run a mile in under 8 minutes by the start of the season. I recommend that girls alternate distance and sprints five to six days a week from May through August and that they run a timed mile every week to chart their progress.

Distance running. At the high school level, the girls should do a mile warm-up, then a harder mile, then about a half-mile cool-down on their distance days. Younger players who start in junior leagues as fourth and fifth graders should get into the habit of easy jogging, working up to a mile, while learning how to stretch. (Many new field hockey players already have experience in other sports, especially soccer.)

Sprint work. Run 4 × 100 yards on a track, or better yet on the field. Then do 4 × 50 and 4 × 25. Finally, do one more 100, timing yourself to see if you can still run fast at the end of a workout. Or, on a track, start by jogging one lap, a 400, then alternate sprinting and jogging the straightaway, about 100, for a mile to a mile and a half. Time your runs to mark progress and work up to sprinting a full 400. Young players should start with a few repetitions at a modest pace and work their way up.

Competitive edge. If you're in shape and can come flying at the ball, you'll make an opposing player think twice about responding when they see how fast you're moving.

Injury prevention. If youngsters have strong legs and are in good shape, injuries such as pulled hamstring and quadriceps muscles, ankle injuries, and shin pain can be reduced or even prevented.

Pushing the pace. Many of our athletes who train diligently are able to run under 7 minutes for the mile time trial, with the fastest girl close to 6 minutes. Midfielders, whose position requires the most running, are usually our fittest athletes.

FOOTBALL: COACH KEN POTTER

> *Credentials: Potter's Jesuit High team of Portland won the Oregon state finals in 2000, 2005, and 2006, and in the last decade the Crusaders have dominated the Metro League with six undefeated seasons. Counting junior varsity and freshman players, he carries a team of 200 in a school with 600 boys and 1,100 students overall. One out of every three boys plays football.*

Running commitment. I encourage our players, as well as all high school athletes, to play multiple sports. In the spring, I want our boys out for tennis, golf, baseball, or track. In the off-season, I want the boys focused on running, primarily for quickness and explosiveness. Likewise, young kids should play as many sports as possible. Not just football but also soccer, racquetball, basketball, or lacrosse. If it's basketball, don't play half-court. Go full-court, getting as much running as possible. In the winter, many of our players are in a CYO basketball league.

Distance running. At the start of the season in late August, we conduct a timed 3-mile run. It's for endurance and team bonding. It's a cross-country-style run on school grounds. Linemen have to do it in 30 minutes; for everyone else, the standard is 25 minutes (8:20 per mile). Before the summer, I give the team a training calendar. Start with a mile twice a week and build to 2 to 3 miles. By the time of our time trial, they should be doing 4 to 6 miles a week.

Sprint work. Twice a week in the summer, do a combination of 20s, 40s, 50s, and 100s. I encourage sprinting hills too.

Competitive edge. During the season, we don't need a lot of separate running because the boys are going full tilt at practice. Still, once a week, on Mondays, we run hills. On a small hill of 15 yards with about a 5 percent incline, we run 15 minutes of repeats, emphasizing high knee action. It's about 20 reps.

Injury prevention. Hill-strengthened players who have developed the quadriceps muscles and hip flexors will reduce injury risk, especially with the nagging little injuries that frequently occur.

Pushing the pace. In the winter, we have a twice-weekly, 45-minute conditioning session with stretching, sprints, and plyometrics drills for whoever shows up.

GYMNASTICS: COACH VALENTINO MOUTAFOV

Credentials: Moutafov is a coach in gymnastics and acrobatics at Scottsdale Gymnastics in Scottsdale, Arizona, and other facilities. Moutafov, who competed in acrobatics in his native Bulgaria, works with all levels, from beginner to elite.

Running commitment. We do track-and-field-style drills and what I call "modified endurance." I can modify the concepts to meet the athletes' personal needs. Recreational kids come for an hour's practice. Elite team members train for two to four hours daily.

Distance running. The longest runs are 10 minutes around the gym as a daily warm-up. Longer running is not relevant to the gymnast.

Sprint work. We do a series of shuttle runs for endurance. You sprint, pick up something, run back. I incorporate jumps plus sideways and backward running. This work enables an athlete to sustain a high-intensity, two-minute floor exercise routine.

Competitive edge. We do long-striding drills with knees up, alternating high right knee, then high left, along with butt kicks in which we extend the legs back. They also walk heel-to-toe to strengthen the feet, which take a pounding.

Injury prevention. You must target all muscle areas. The more well-trained athletes who have muscular balance will suffer less injury.

Pushing the pace. To add speed to leg movement, the youngsters lie on their backs while spinning their legs in a fast, circular, bicycle-style motion. Also, we push mats around the floor at top speed and the kids run with a partner holding them back using a bungee around the hips. The legs are always working in gymnastics routines.

LACROSSE: COACH CHUCK RUEBLING

Credentials: The 2007 squad of Ruebling, the assistant headmaster and lacrosse coach at the all-boys Delbarton School in Morristown, New Jersey, was ranked sixth in the nation. That same season Delbarton was the state group winner in the non-public A division and Ruebling was named state Coach of the Year.

Running commitment. You have to be in exceptional physical condition to perform throughout a contest. The field is 110 yards by 60 yards. There are 12-minute quarters. The goalie and some other players among the ten starters play the entire 48 minutes. In girls' lacrosse, which is growing, they play two 25-minute halves but with running time.

Distance running. We expect kids to be in shape in March when spring practice starts. I hold a 1-mile time trial looking for a time of 7 minutes or better. The athletes have to prepare with several weeks of training.

Sprint work. The emphasis is on short bursts with recovery, and for all youngsters I recommend sprinting the length of the field (110 yards) while jogging the width (60 yards). Start with 5 reps and build to 10 three times a week.

Competitive edge. For continuous movement that simulates the stop-and-start rhythm of a game, do 20-yard sprints ten times back and forth without stopping, 20 sprints overall. We like to see players do this set in under two minutes. The change in direction builds opposing muscle groups.

Injury prevention. The fitter players have less injury and missed time.

Pushing the pace. To set high standards and motivate the athletes, everything we do is timed. We do a set of ten to twenty 50-yard sprints, each one to be run in under 7 seconds, with a 10-second recovery. Any sprint clocking above 7 seconds is not counted. Younger kids, say age 10, should aim for a time of 9 to 10 seconds with a 20-second recovery.

NORDIC SKIING: COLLEGE ATHLETE BEN TRUE

Credentials: True, both a cross-country runner and cross-country skier for years, is a six-time Heptagonal conference winner on the Dartmouth track and cross-country squads and a member of the Big Green team that won the NCAA nordic skiing championship in 2007.

Running commitment. Young skiers should do plenty of hill running on cross-country terrain. The idea is to push the uphills, in an explosive manner like bounding, while running relaxed on the flats and downhills. The bounding style will develop the "pop" in your legs necessary in cross-country skiing. Running benefits all three cross-country techniques—double poling, striding, and classical.

Distance running. For hill repetitions, pick a hill of medium length and steepness, and run up for about 15 to 20 seconds, using the downhill as recovery. If the hill is too long or too steep, you won't be able to run with good form for long.

Sprint work. Sprints are not a must in cross-country skiing, which boasts some of the world's fittest athletes based on aerobic capacity. However, some Nordic skiers specialize in sprinting and do more interval work than distance.

Competitive edge. I advocate "moosehoofs," a Scandinavian term that means running on undulating terrain. Do a 30-minute run on a cross-country course in which you go hard on the uphills while holding a moderate pace (more than a jog) on the flats and downhills.

Injury prevention. Running and skiing ideally complement each other, providing tremendous year-round aerobic benefit with reduced pounding of the body.

Pushing the pace. Occasionally switch off hills to flat runs at a fast pace to maintain quick leg turnover.

SOFTBALL: COACH DEBBIE SCHWARTZ

Credentials: In twenty seasons of coaching at New Jersey state power Toms River East, Schwartz, also the school's supervisor of health and physical education, has amassed 380 career wins. As an athlete who starred in field hockey, Schwartz is a member of the Ocean County and Toms River Halls of Fame.

Running commitment. All of our running is based on injury prevention. The girls have to start the season in March with muscles ready to work.

Distance running. In January, I give the girls a six-week program that entails building up to a 1.5-to-2-mile run. They start with a half mile three days a week. I'm not worried about time, just completing the distance. Once the season begins, they run a half mile every day. Younger players can do easy jogging. Keep it informal, keep the kids moving. Don't call it "training." Have the girls play running games on the infield within the bases.

Sprint work. Prior to the season, the girls run sprints, like sets of 60s or 100s.

Competitive edge. We do a lot of agility training on the run, like butt kicks and plyometrics drills. Working on these agility skills can prepare you for competition and prevent injury.

Injury prevention. Fitter kids have fewer injuries. We want to avoid pulled muscles, which can keep a player sidelined for up to ten days.

Pushing the pace. We have a three-month season from early March to early June. The rest of the year, I urge the girls to work on weights and other forms of strength training.

SOCCER: COACH FRANK DIXON

Credentials: Now in his eighteenth season coaching the Carmel High girls soccer team in Carmel, Indiana, Dixon's Greyhounds have won ten state crowns and in 2002 were ranked number one in the country in two national soccer polls.

Running commitment. In soccer, you can't get away with being anything less than a fit runner, especially on the high school level with 80-minute games (40-minute halves, running time). We do many forms of running that are fun so athletes look forward to it.

Distance running. To measure fitness prior to school, we hold a 2-mile time trial in early August. Our goal is under 16 minutes. Most of our girls play club soccer and are in shape throughout the year. I also recommend that they run spring track, a nice crossover sport that works well in conjunction with club soccer practices. Younger players, from 7 to 13, do not need much structured running. Running 20 minutes three times a week, in a fun way with friends, would be sufficient. Make a game out of it; run some relays.

Sprint work. We do a lot of running-style drills with the ball. Occasionally, we do a sprint set like 10 × 120 yards in 17 to 20 seconds each with a jog back to the start in between.

Competitive edge. Line up with a partner and pass the ball back and forth while running the field. Or sprint while dribbling or passing the ball up the field, and sprint back without the ball. Or run the field with a partner in which one player throws the ball and the other heads it. These drills are forms of "hidden running" that work on skills and conditioning at the same time.

Injury prevention. We include backward running to build hamstring strength, so that the hamstring muscles will achieve balance with the quadriceps muscles, reducing risk of knee injury.

Pushing the pace. Soccer and running are closely allied, and in the same fall season I have had some athletes do the two sports simultaneously. One was an individual state cross-country champion; others have played on both state soccer and cross-country championship squads.

SWIMMING: COACH MIKE SULLIVAN

Credentials: Sullivan has been coaching state power Christian Brothers Academy (CBA), an all-boys' school in Lincroft, New Jersey, for nineteen years, and all nineteen years the Colts have won the Shore Conference, the largest and most competitive conference in the state.

Running commitment. In swimming, it's essential to develop the cardiovascular system. This applies to all strokes and all distances.

Distance running. Swimming is an oxygen-deprivation sport, and cross-training is the way to go. Many competitors swim year-round on club teams and YMCA teams in addition to the school team. If you're in the water three or four times a week, I would advise running a mile or so the other three days. Young kids can start with a quarter mile and work up to a mile.

Sprint work. This does not apply in swimming, where endurance is crucial.

Competitive edge. For dry-land conditioning, we also derive cardiovascular benefit from circuit training in the weight room, doing low weights with high reps for 30 seconds at each of fifteen stations.

Injury prevention. A fit swimmer tires less easily, maintaining proper form in the pool to reduce risk of shoulder injury. In meets, a high school swimmer may do as many as four events in an hour.

Pushing the pace. Many top runners start out in swimming. American mile record-holder Alan Webb is among the notable examples. At CBA, we currently have a young swimmer who also runs cross-country and has excellent potential in both sports.

TENNIS: COACH PAT ETCHEBERRY

> *Credentials: Etcheberry, a fitness trainer in tennis at Saddlebrook Resort in Wesley Chapel, Florida, coached many top pros in their early years, including Pete Sampras and Jim Courier. At Etcheberry Sports Performance, his client list includes professional athletes in many sports.*

Running commitment. Tennis is a running sport. Look at a match. You have to be quick, able to perform with fast recovery. There are only 20 to 25 seconds' rest between points.

Distance running. Track-and-field-style interval running is the key, but it's always important to do a warm-up mile prior to sprints.

Sprint work. The nature of intervals depends somewhat on the style of player. Jim Courier had to work harder on the court—do more running—than Pete Sampras, a power player with a big serve, to win a point. I would give Courier rigorous intervals like three sets of 8 × 100 meters with 30 seconds' rest between sprints and a 2-minute rest between sets. Or 15 × 200s with a 60-second rest between runs. Sampras, on the other hand, would do 20s, 40s, 50s. He ran less on the court. I would give him two sets of 10 × 40s, finishing with a set of 100s. Both men rose to become number one in the world.

Competitive edge. Fitness can make up for lack of skills. Courier, as well as Thomas Muster, are examples. They were not the most talented players but worked harder than others and could grind out long matches to win championships.

Injury prevention. The legs take a pounding, especially the knee and the muscles around it, the hamstrings and quadriceps. A well-conditioned athlete can absorb more shock to the legs, thereby reducing the likelihood of injury.

Pushing the pace. A long match, like five sets for men lasting several hours, might seem to require aerobic conditioning, but what's really called for is "speed endurance." You must move fast and recover over and over again. The fittest tennis players could run a very fast 100 meters and repeat it several times with little rest.

VOLLEYBALL: COACH LISA ARCE

> *Credentials: In 2007, Arce's Mira Costa High girls team in Manhattan Beach, California, had a 37–0 record and was ranked number one in the country by Prepvolleyball.com.*

Running commitment. Running is important to develop the stamina to sustain a long season. Volleyball is a fall sport with matches every week. A game typically takes about 20 minutes, and in a three-out-of-five contest there would be about an hour of play. But volleyball is an anaerobic sport with explosive movement. A lot of volleyball is reacting, and you need the strength and stamina from the first jump to the last jump of a match.

Distance running. We do 2 miles at least two to three days a week. The girls should develop the ability to run 2 miles in 14 minutes, and no slower than 16 minutes. Occasionally we do a timed mile to check their pace and as a gut check. The younger freshmen start out at around 18 minutes for 2 miles. Kids starting in volleyball around age 10 should do 5-minute runs (a little more than a half mile) a few days a week.

Sprint work. We do sprints three days a week in the gym, in which three volleyball courts fill the size of the arena. For example, stand at the end line, run to the end of the first court and back; then run to the end of the second court and back; then run to the end of the third court and back. We do many variations, including backward running, sideways running, high-knee running, changing directions throughout. We go nonstop for about 20 minutes, doing forty to fifty short sprints.

Competitive edge. In the off-season, in spring, we have a program in which we alternate sprints and jumping rope (for agility) one day with running a mile and a half on the track plus stadium steps the other day.

Injury prevention. To minimize shin splits, our most common ailment, we do some body lunges, three sets of 12 on each leg, twice a week. Core strength, which helps with balance, is also important in reducing injury.

Pushing the pace. Volleyball is popular in our area and most of our girls play on clubs in the off-season. They do at least a two-hour practice three days a week, helping them stay in shape year-round.

WRESTLING: COACH TIM FLYNN

Credentials: Flynn coaches the wrestling team at Edinboro University in Pennsylvania. His squad placed ninth and eighth, respectively, in the 2006 and 2007 NCAA championships.

Running commitment. In college, a match is seven minutes; in high school it's six minutes. That's a long time on the mat, and it takes a base of cardiovascular conditioning to get through a bout. A fit wrestler can overcome lack of size or skill to prevail.

Distance running. When school starts, we do a five-week program of sprints and distance three to four days a week, along with wrestling practice. For distance, we start with a 3-mile run and work up to 5 miles and longer.

Sprint work. We do a weekly sprint workout on the track: 200s, 400s, and 800s that total 1.5 to 3 miles. We also sprint up and down hills. Young wrestlers doing hills should walk down to avoid stress on the knees.

Competitive edge. In the gym, we do sprints for 24 minutes, running the court in a number of variations with brief rest.

Injury prevention. A tired wrestler increases injury risk to the knees, calves, and quadriceps muscles.

Pushing the pace. We also do "buddy carries," in which pairs of athletes alternate carrying one another on their backs for about a hundred steps at a time for a mile out, then a mile back, 2 miles in all. It's good for wrestlers' legs.

Appendix

Running Events Nationwide

Following is a sampling of children's running programs and events, with assistance from Running USA youth program coordinator Linda Honikman, runningusa.org.

 EVENTS BY STATE

Alabama

Mercedes Kids Marathon, 1 mile, Birmingham, February.
    www.mercedesmarathon.com
Autumn Chase Fun Run, 1 mile, Huntsville, September.
    www.huntsvilletrackclub.org

Arkansas

Andy Allison's Super Kids Run, 1 mile, Arkadelphia, April.
    www.dltmultisport.com

Arizona

Phoenix Children's Hospital Kids Rock, 1 mile, Tempe, January.
www.kidsrockaz.com

California

Great Race of Agoura, 1 mile, Agoura Hills, April.
www.greatraceofagoura.com

Junior Carlsbad, 1 mile, Carlsbad, April. www.eliteracing.com

Keebler's Kids Marathon Mile, 1 mile, Carlsbad, January.
www.sdmarathon.com

Kids Hot to Trot, 1 mile, Dana Point, November.
www.justrun.org

LA84 Run 4 Fun, 2K (1.25 miles), Los Angeles, December.
www.la84foundation.org

Spirit Run, 1 mile, Newport Beach, March.
www.kinaneevents.com

Oceanside Turkey Trot, 1 mile, Oceanside, November.
www.kinaneevents.com

Heart and Sole Kids Run, 1 mile, Salinas, May. www.justrun.org

Union-Tribune Kids Magic Mile, 1 mile, San Diego, May.
www.inmotionevents.com

Spreckels 4th of July Kids Run, 1 mile, Spreckels, July.
www.justrun.org

Dinosaur Dash Kids Run, 2K (1.25 miles), Tustin, November.
www.dinosaurdash.net

Disney Family Fun Run, 5K (3.1 miles), Anaheim, August.
www.disneyenduranceseries.com

Childrens Hospital Los Angeles Kids on the Run, 5K (3.1 miles)
and 10K (6.2 miles), Los Angeles, February.
www.kidsontherun.net

Colorado

Bolder Boulder Middle School Challenge, 10K (6.2 miles),
Boulder, May. www.bolderboulder.com
Cherry Creek Sneak Student Sprint, 1 mile, Denver, April.
www.ccsneak.com
Colorado Kids Marathon, 1 mile, Denver, May.
www.coloradocolfaxmarathon.org
McDonald's Mile Kids Race, 1 mile, Denver, October.
www.denvermarathon.com

Connecticut

Greater Danbury Kids Run, .5 mile, Danbury, April.
www.jbsports.com
Hartford Kids/ING Run for Something Better Mile, 1 mile,
Hartford, October. www.hartfordmarathon.com
New Haven Children's Run, 800 meters, New Haven,
September. www.jbsports.com

District of Columbia

Race for the Cure/DC Kids, 1K (.6 mile), Washington, April.
www.nationalraceforthecure.org
Cherry Blossom Kids Run, 1K (.6 mile), Washington, April.
www.cherryblossom.org

Florida

Adidas Junior River Run, 1 mile, Jacksonville, March.
www.1stplacesports.com
Pensacola Kids Marathon, 1.2 miles, Pensacola, February.
www.pensacolamarathon.com

Junior Gasparilla Classic, 800 meters, Tampa, February.
www.tampabayrun.com

St. Pete Beach Kids Races, 1 mile, St. Petersburg, January.
www.motionsportsmanagement.com

Bay to Bay Kids Races, 1 mile, St. Petersburg, March.
www.motionsportsmanagement.com

Kids Read 'n' Run Marathon, 1.2 miles, West Palm Beach,
December. www.marathonpb.com

Smile Mile, 1 mile, Winter Park, February. www.trackshack.com

Georgia

Peachtree Junior, 3K (1.9 miles), Atlanta, May.
www.atlantatrackclub.org

Idaho

St. Alphonsus Capitol Classic, 1 mile, Boise, June.
www.saintalphonsus.org

Illinois

Park Forest Scenic Kids Run, 800 meters. Park Forest, Illinois,
September. www.villageofparkforest.com

Iowa

Alcoa Junior Bix 7, .7 mile, Davenport, July. www.bix7.com

Children's Center at Mercy Kids Run, .5 mile, Des Moines,
October. www.desmoinesmarathon.com

Maine

Beach to Beacon Youth Run, 1K (.6 mile), Cape Elizabeth,
    August. www.beach2beacon.org

Maryland

Kids Fun Run, .33 mile, Baltimore, October.
    www.thebaltimoremarathon.com
Darcars Young Run, 1 mile, Rockville, October. www.mcrrc.org

Massachusetts

Great Bear Run, 400 meters, Needham, May.
    www.needhamtrack.org
Heartbreak Hill International Youth Race, 1 mile, Newton,
    April. www.newtonpride.org

Michigan

Blue Care Network Kids Run, .5 mile, Ann Arbor, May.
    www.dexterannarborrun.com
Crim Kids Classic, .5 mile, Flint, May. www.crim.org
Crim Teddy Bear Trot, .25 mile, Flint, August. www.crim.org
Junior River Bank Run, 1 mile, Grand Rapids, May.
    www.53riverbankrun.com

Minnesota

Whipper Snapper, 400 meters, Duluth, June.
    www.grandmasmarathon.com
Park Point Youth Races, 1 mile, Duluth, July.
    www.grandmasmarathon.com

Medtronic Twin Cities Marathon Kids Races, .5 and 1 mile,
   Minneapolis, October. www.mtcmarathon.org
Medtronic Twin Cities Kids Cross-Country Run, 3K (1.9 miles),
   Minneapolis, May. www.mtcmarathon.org

Montana

Huffing for Stuffing, 1K (.6 mile), Bozeman, November.
   www.huffingforstuffing.com
Missoula Kids Marathon, 1.2 miles, Missoula, July.
   www.runwildmissoula.org

Nebraska

Great Pumpkin Run, 1 mile, Lincoln, October.
   www.lincolnrun.org
KFRX Mayor's Run for Children, 1 mile, Lincoln, May.
   www.lincolnrun.org

New Jersey

Spring Lake 5 Kids' Races, 25 yards to .25 mile, Spring Lake,
   May. www.springlake5.org

New Mexico

Run for the Zoo, 1 mile, Albuquerque, May.
   www.bioparksociety.org
Sun Healthcare Duke City, 1K (.6 mile), October.
   www.dukecitymarathon.com

New York

Freihofer's Run for Kids, .5 mile, Albany, May.
www.freihofersrun.com
Adidas Run for the Parks Kids Run, .5 mile, New York, April.
www.nyrr.org
Syracuse Festival of Races, 400 meters, Syracuse, October.
www.festivalofraces.com
Utica National Insurance Youth Run, 1 mile, Utica, July.
www.boilermaker.com

North Dakota

Scheels Fargo Kids Run, 1 mile, Fargo, May.
www.fargomarathon.com

Ohio

Road Runner Akron Kids Run, 1K (.6 mile), Akron, September.
www.akronmarathon.org
Flying Piglet, 5K (3.1 miles), Cincinnati, May.
www.flyingpigmarathon.com

Oregon

Eugene Kids Marathon, 1 mile, Eugene, May.
www.eugenemarathon.com
Marafun Kids Run, 2 miles, Portland, October.
www.portlandmarathon.org
Awesome 3000, 3K (1.9 miles), Salem, May.
www.skeducationfoundation.org

Pennsylvania

Philadelphia Children's Run, 1 mile, Philadelphia, September.
www.runphilly.com
Junior Great Race, 1 mile, Pittsburgh, September.
www.rungreatrace.com
Broad Street Fun Miler and Diaper Derby, 1 mile, Philadelphia,
May. www.broadstreetrun.com

Rhode Island

CVS Caremark Downtown Kids Run, 100 meters, Providence,
September. www.cvsdowntown5k.com

South Carolina

Junior Kids Cooper River Bridge Run, .25 mile, Charleston,
April. www.bridgerun.com

Tennessee

Little 8s Kids Runs, 800 meters, Kingsport, July.
www.crazy8s.org
Knoxville Marathon Kids Run, 1.2 miles, Knoxville, March.
www.knoxvillemarathon.com
Knoxville Kids Road Mile, 1 mile, Knoxville, May.
www.ktcyouthathletics.org
YMCA Country Music Kids Marathon, 1 mile, Nashville, April.
www.cmmarathon.com

Texas

Austin American-Statesman Junior 'Dillo, 1 mile, Austin,
March. www.statesman.com

Cowtown Kids Run, 5K (3.1 miles), Fort Worth, February.
www.cowtownmarathon.org
Texas Children's Hospital Kids' Fun Run, 3K (1.9 miles),
Houston, January. www.chevronhoustonmarathon.com

Virginia

Marine Corps Marathon Healthy Kids Fun Run, 1 mile,
Arlington, October. www.marinemarathon.com
First Market Mile, 1 mile, Richmond, April.
www.sportsbackers.com
Richmond Times-Dispatch Kids Run, 1 mile, November.
www.richmondmarathon.com
Shamrock Sportsfest Smile Mile Final, 1 mile, Virginia Beach,
March. www.shamrockmarathon.com

Washington

America's Kids Run, 1 mile, Spokane, April.
www.americaskidsrun.org
Seattle Kids Marathon, 1.2 miles, Seattle, November.
www.seattlemarathon.org
Fit for Bloomsday Run, 12K (7.4 miles), Spokane, May.
www.bloomsdayrun.org

Wisconsin

Guardian Kids Fun Run, .5 mile, Appleton, September.
www.foxcitiesmarathon.org
Bellin 10K Kids for Running, 10K (6.2 miles), Bellin, June.
www.bellinrun.com
Wisconsin Public Service Kids Power, 800 meters, Green Bay,
May. www.cellcomgreenbaymarathon.com

▶ YOUTH RUNNING PROGRAMS AND RACE SERIES

Big Sur Marathon Just Run Program, Monterey County,
    California, and elsewhere, www.justrun.org
Brockton Kids Road Race Series, 2.2 miles, Brockton,
    Massachusetts, www.kidsroadraces.org
Colgate Women's Games, New York City area indoor track
    series, Brooklyn and Manhattan, www.colgategames.com
CrimFit Youth Programs, Flint, Michigan, www.crim.org
Disney's Kids Races, Lake Buena Vista, Florida,
    www.disneyenduranceseries.com
Duluth Wednesday Night at the Races, 1 mile, Duluth,
    Minnesota, www.grandmasmarathon.com
Feelin' Good Mileage Club, Michigan schools and elsewhere,
    www.fitnessfinders.com
Fit for Bloomsday, Spokane, Washington area schoolchildren,
    www.bloomsdayrun.org
Fit for Life Program, central Virginia schoolchildren,
    www.sportsbackers.com
Fit Girls, girls in Medfield, Massachusetts, area and spreading
    elsewhere, www.fitgirls.org
Freehold Area Running Club Kids' Summer Nights, summer
    race series in central New Jersey, www.farcnj.com
Girls on the Run, girls 8–13 nationwide, www.girlsontherun.org
GO! St. Louis Family Fitness Program, St. Louis area school
    children, www.gostlouis.org
ING Run for Something Better, Miami area schoolchildren,
    www.ingmiamimarathon.com
Intermountain Kids Marathon, Utah schoolchildren,
    www.seattlemarathon.org
Many Milers, Vermont schoolchildren, www.runvermont.org
Marathon Kids, schoolchildren in Texas and elsewhere,
    www.marathonkids.org

Medtronic Twin Cities Marathon Program, Minnesota schoolchildren, www.mtcmarathon.org

Motivating Movement Through Marathoning, for Cleveland, Ohio, area schoolchildren, www.clevelandmarathon.com

Nike 5K for Kids, eight cities nationwide, www.nike5kforkids.com

New York Road Runners Foundation, schoolchildren in New York City and elsewhere, www.nyrr.org

Run for Orange County Kids, southern California children, www.ocmarathon.com

Run SFM Youth Outreach Program, at-risk San Francisco area youth, www.runsfm.com

Students Run LA, at-risk middle and high school students in Los Angeles, www.srla.org

Students Run Philly Style, at-risk middle and high school students in Philadelphia, www.nncc.us

▶ NATIONAL YOUTH TRACK SERIES

Amateur Athletic Union Junior Olympics, www.aaujrogames.org

Hershey's Track and Field Games, www.hersheystrackandfield.com

USA Track and Field Junior Olympics, www.usatf.org

USA Track and Field Youth Championships, www.usatf.org

▶ GRANT PROGRAMS

Road Runners Clubs of America Kids Run the Nation, www.rrca.org

Robert Wood Johnson Foundation, www.rwjf.org

Saucony Run for Good Foundation, www.sauconyrunforgood.com

USA Track and Field Foundation, www.usatf.org

Acknowledgments

S ince watching young runners in action is always a thrill for me, putting this book together was pure joy. While seeking the best advice on running for children and teenagers, I put myself in close quarters with young runners of all ages, from toddlers and little kids to the preteens and teens I often see at middle school and high school events. I thank the young runner community at large: all the many youngsters and parents, teachers and coaches, race organizers, doctors, and sports medicine specialists, for welcoming my inquiries, and visits, with open arms and a shared commitment to helping young people enjoy the countless benefits of healthy running.

In particular, the following people were most gracious in giving me their time and expertise: Isabel Keeley and the Freehold Area Running Club in Monmouth County, New Jersey; Richard Dexter and the staff of Lynbrook Elementary School in Springfield, Virginia; Dr. Brenda Armstrong of the Durham Striders youth track club and Duke University Medical School in Durham, North Carolina; Frank Davis of the Durham Striders; coach and teacher Calliope Anthanasakos and the staff at Intermediate School 30 in Brooklyn; coaches and special education teachers

Caolan Sinisi and Glenn Odato of Marlboro Middle School in Monmouth County, New Jersey; coach and teacher Eric Hill of St. Bernard's School in Manhattan; coach and teacher Steve Sloan of Public School 102 in Harlem; Cliff Sperber (executive director) and Paola Baptiste (program manager) of the New York Road Runners Foundation; Linda Honikman of Running USA; and Pat Mantone of Marlboro Elementary School in Monmouth County, the teacher most responsible for the compelling story of Danny Mininsohn, the autistic boy in my community who runs.

I also thank Danny's parents, Anne Marie and Eric, for allowing me into their lives, to follow Danny's running and join in their excitement as Danny continued his remarkable progress in middle school track and cross-country. Danny's primary physician, Dr. Susan E. Levy of Children's Hospital of Philadelphia, has been a great help in enabling me to better understand autism and aspects of Danny's development. And I thank Danny himself for the privilege of becoming his running partner and friend. He has taught me a lot.

There are many other authorities and people involved with children and teenage running who offered important ideas. They include Molly Barker, founder of Girls on the Run; Steven Blair, Ph.D., professor of exercise science, epidemiology, and biostatistics at the University of South Carolina; Dr. Susan Carter, a gynecological surgeon, and high school cross-country coach, in Greeley, Colorado; Mike Dove of the Just Run program in the Monterey Peninsula of California; Joel Fish, Ph.D., director of the Center for Sports Psychology in Philadelphia; Coach Bob Glover, who directs the New York Road Runners Foundation City Sports For Kids Program; Michigan State University sports psychologist Daniel Gould, Ph.D., director of the school's Institute for Study of Youth Sports; Dr. Kenneth Indahl, a podiatrist and Ironman triathlete in Wall Township, New Jersey; Jay Marden, principal of Carmel River Elementary School in California, and a former Olympic Trials track competitor; Rick Nealis, race director of the Marine Corps Marathon Healthy Kids Fun Run; Sean Neihoff, a PE teacher at Eagle View Elementary School in Fairfax County, Virginia; Russ Pate, Ph.D., professor of exercise science at the University of South Carolina, and a former Olympic Trials marathon competitor; Lizzie Peterson, children's footwear buyer at Playmakers in Okemos, Michigan; Dr. Stephen G. Rice, director of the Jersey Shore Sports Medicine Center at University Medical Center in Neptune, New Jersey; Dr. Bill Roberts of Minneapolis, past president of the American College of Sports Medicine and medical director of the Twin Cities Marathon; Dr. Michael E. Sargent of the Department of Orthopedics at Vermont School of Medicine; Dr. Mona Shangold, director of the Center for Women's Health and Sports Gynecology in Philadelphia; Dr. Jennifer Sluder, a pediatrician at Childrens Hospital Los Angeles who's involved with a number of running programs; Dr. Angela Smith, an orthopedist at Children's Hospital of Philadelphia; and the "world's busiest coach," Bill Sumner, who counsels up to 2,000 runners of all ages on a weekly basis in southern California.

My appreciation also goes to the coaches of non-running sports who were generous with their expertise, covered in chapter 14: Lisa Arce (volleyball), Steven Berlack (alpine skiing), Frank Dixon (soccer), Pat Etcheberry (tennis), Tim Flynn (wrestling), Don Landolphi (baseball), Valentino Moutafov (gymnastics), Evan Pickman (basketball), Ken Potter (football), Chuck Ruebling (lacrosse), Debbie Schwartz (softball), Mike Sullivan (swimming), and Tisha Werner (field hockey). And to the athlete who helped with alpine skiing, Ben True of Dartmouth.

Part of the joy in writing *Young Runners* stems from the support of the Touchstone Fireside team at Simon & Schuster, led by my editor, Zachary Schisgal, whose guidance has helped make this book something I'm proud to hold in my hands. I am most grateful to my literary agent, Richard Curtis, who can always tell when a writer needs a boost to marshal creative energy.

For both editorial judgment and a shoulder to lean on, I can never do better than my wife, Andrea, a teacher whose high standards and unrelenting work ethic show me the way. We look forward to sharing in the thrill of seeing our grandchildren take their first laps around the track.

Index